Contents

List of contributors

Colin Beacock MA Cert. Ed, RNLD, RGN
RCN Advisor in Learning Disabilities, London, UK

Peter Eldridge BA MA
Joint Research Officer, New Possibilities NHS Trust, Witham, Essex, UK, and Department of Health and Human Sciences, University of Essex, Colchester, Essex, UK

Brian Kay RNLD RNT Cert. Ed (FE) Dip. Phil
Director of Development, Choice Support, East Dulwich, London, UK

Revd Jeanne Males BA, MPhil, PhD, AFBPsS
Assistant Curate, St. Mary the Blessed Virgin, Addington, Surrey

Anne Markwick BA(Hons) RNLD
Director of Nursing and Workforce Development, Hertfordshire Partnership Trust, St Albans, UK

Brian McGinnis BA OBE
Special Advisor Mencap, London, UK

Alan Parrish OBE RNLD RGN
Former Learning Disabilities Advisor, Royal College of Nursing, London, UK

Sue Read MA (Community Care: Mental Handicap), RNMH, Cert. Ed (FE), Certificate in bereavement studies
Lecturer, Keele University, Department of Nursing and Midwifery, City General Hospital, Stoke on Trent, Staffordshire, UK

David Sines BSc(Hons) PhD RN RNMH RMN RNT PGCTHE ILTM FRCN FRSA
Professor of Community Health Nursing and Dean of the Faculty of Health, South Bank University, London, UK

John Stagg RNMH Dip. H.E
Clinical Nurse Specialist, East Specialist Health Care Team, Hawthorn Lodge, Moorgreen Hospital, Southampton, UK

Lesley Styring RNMS MEd DPSN
Nurse Consultant-Respite, Community Health Sheffield, UK

Foreword

I regard it as both a pleasure and a privilege to have been invited to produce the Foreword for this innovative and thought-provoking text. Over the past three decades I have been personally associated with the lives of people with learning disabilities, their carers and their professional supporters. Together, we have witnessed many changes, which overall have resulted in the enhancement of the rights, status and position of people with learning disabilities. However, as this insightful text will bear witness, the journey towards meaningful inclusion within society is far from concluded.

Endorsement of this sentiment was provided by the Government in March 2001, when it acknowledged the need to provide further investment and strategic commitment to improving the lives of people with learning disabilities. The result was *Valuing people*, the Government's new strategy for people with learning disability, which in the words of the Prime Minister noted that 'some people find themselves pushed to the margins of society…almost all encounter prejudice, bullying, insensitive treatment and discrimination at some time in their lives'. *Valuing people* (Department of Health, 2001) presents a vision that aims to build a society in which all people with disabilities can participate as equal citizens.

The Government has outlined a comprehensive strategy based on listening to service users, their carers and supporters and to its credit it has done so in the absence of a substantive or robust quantitative evidence base. However, as with this inspiring text, the richness of debate and a range of ensuing pragmatic recommendations for change have been informed by personal testimony and experience provided by those people who have direct insight into learning disability and into the provision of care and support for this client group.

It is the book's reliance on the inclusion of case studies and informed vision that sets it apart from other books. It outlines the many changes that have taken place in the public perception and acceptance of people with learning disabilities, and in the provision of innovative and pragmatic service responses and solutions, designed to promote inclusion.

Overall the text provides a rationale for a new 'rights-based vision' that incorporates the principles of independence, choice and user participation. However, such bold principles have so often failed to penetrate the actual lives of service users, many of whom have been denied the right to free expression of opinion, choice and self-determination. It is therefore encouraging to note that the contributors to this text have adopted a thematic approach to exploring a range of challenging subjects that together, impact on the perceived quality of life experience for service users. Profoundly important ethically challenging topics such as bereavement and loss, abuse, sexuality and spirituality have been thoroughly analysed and are accompanied by insight into the issues that confront service users from their own perspectives. A range of practical solutions and strategies for self-help accompanies each topic.

The text also confronts key issues such as the provision of responsive public health and health promotion services, the management of service transition, dual diagnosis, the provision of residential and community day services and the educational support required by carers and support staff to effectively respond to the needs of service users.

The book offers an exciting package that provides an excellent complement to the government's agenda for change. Its main strength is the provision of a pragmatic vision for the future based on human rights, self-determination, inclusion and equity. It also places users of services at the centre of service monitoring and change.

It is my contention that the realisation of excellence in the design and delivery of responsive services relies upon the principle that service users, their carers and support staff require and deserve mutual recognition as key stakeholders in the development and implementation of future policy imperatives. This text aims to ensure that this principle becomes a reality. Some may challenge the 'realism' of the authors' suggestions and recommendations, but there is one statement that cannot be challenged — they are all feasible, and evidence exists to suggest that further investment and commitment to improving the diverse and varied life opportunities of people with learning disabilities will result in a more fulfilling future for us all.

David Sines

REFERENCES   Department of Health 2001 Valuing people: a new strategy for learning disability for the 21st century. The Stationery Office, London

Preface

This book will take its place amongst the many texts aimed at professionals working with people with learning disabilities. However, it is set apart from other mainstream texts in that each chapter is underpinned with a case study or example, in which all names used are fictional, based on the personal experience of the author. This means that each chapter is rooted in reality, based on lived experience and maintains the centrality of the service user. Through this approach the book is able to address a number of key themes.

Acknowledged experts in their respective areas have contributed to the chapters. The diversity of the contributors allows the text to develop its themes through a wide range of situations and shows how central these issues are to this potentially very vulnerable group.

The text is significantly different from other publications in this field in that it has veered away from social policy and the broader contextual issues and concentrated on the lived experience of individuals with learning disabilities and the professionals and others who support them in their daily living.

As the editors we believe that the book will be of value not only to qualified nurses and students undergoing training but it will also be useful for members of a multidisciplinary team and others either central to, or on the fringe of, this field. The chapters are accessible and thought-provoking and provide a diversity of view and experience that will be useful to many. Focusing on the client as a person and tackling the sensitive and challenging issues for service providers, it should stimulate the reader and encourage self-analysis and reflection.

The book is timely in that it complements and supports the publication of the Government's strategy for learning disability for the 21st century, *Valuing people* (Department of Health, 2001), which sets out to eliminate prejudice and discrimination as well as pointing out the situation we needed to change. In a modern civilised society in which everyone should be valued, opportunity has to be given to all citizens to play their part in society. The key is to enable that process and not to disable people.

Back in 1993 (NHS Management Executive, 1993) a person with a learning disability (the person is not named) said, 'You drew a line and put me on one side of it and yourself on the other. Why should I suffer from being on the wrong side of your line?' It's time we erased the line. We hope this book will help.

Anne Markwick
Alan Parrish

St Albans and London 2003

REFERENCES   Department of Health 2001 Valuing people: a new strategy for learning disability for the 21st century (Cm 5086). The Stationery Office, London
National Health Service Management Executive 1993 Learning disabilities. Department of Health, London

Acknowledgements

This book has taken a long time getting to publication. The initial idea and discussions with the authors and the publisher started in 1999.

The experience was new to us both and proved to be exciting, challenging and at times quite frustrating. It also proved to be a larger undertaking than we had initially thought.

It was not in our thinking for the book to be anything other than a useful, practical and thought-provoking publication. Although it has to have an academic base, we wanted much of the writing to record or reflect the real world of the professionals and their relationship and working day with people who have learning disabilities.

We are both grateful to our families, friends and colleagues, who have supported us through this interesting exercise.

We particularly wish to thank sincerely our fellow contributors for their efforts in getting the book to publication.

1 Introduction

Alan Parrish and Anne Markwick

Successive UK governments have had a commitment to improve the health of the nation, and in doing so the focus has been to shift delivery of care from hospitals and institutions into the community. This commitment stretches back to the 1971 White Paper *Better services for the mentally handicapped* (Department of Health and Social Security, 1971) and is confirmed by the community care White Paper *Caring for people* (Department of Health, 1989). These were then supported by two further circulars in October 1992 (Department of Health, 1992a,b). These documents have had a profound effect on some groups of clients/patients and their families and on the way professionals think and practise.

Care for the majority of people starts at home; however, over the years, the alternative for the person with a learning disability was institutional care. In this case, the family and their involvement often became distanced. This problem has been addressed by the reintroduction of clients/patients into a community-based service, generally in a locality nearer to their friends and relatives.

During the 1970s, the values that underpinned the hospital and hostel-style provision for people with a learning disability were questioned by a range of groups and, not least, by the clients themselves. Pressure groups, parents and professionals no longer saw the style and standard of living being provided in a hospital as suitable for the person with a disability. Values that had become outdated, and had placed those being cared for in a subservient position with little or no say in the decisions that affected them each day, were replaced gradually with the individual's right to be heard and have their wishes acted upon. This was a difficult adjustment for many professionals and it was particularly difficult for some parents; it still remains a challenge for some.

The demise of this institutional care model, with a service that often was run for the convenience of staff and not for the benefit of the residents, was followed by a period of both instability and uncertainty. Happily, throughout all the changes, the client group grew in stature and developed with exposure to different and more usual experiences in the community settings. The way that this group of previously oppressed people have grasped the nettle of independence, risk taking and decision making has been a surprise to some and an education to many. The new care models, supported by the new strategy, will allow this process to continue and strengthen, enabling individuals and groups to be, and to feel, truly part of society.

VALUING PEOPLE   The first strategy for learning disabilities to be produced by government in 30 years, *Valuing people*, is designed to address social discrimination and exclusion (Department of Health, 2001). The document strategy is based on four principles:

- civil rights
- independence
- choice
- inclusion.

It is an exciting, challenging and well thought out strategy. If its objectives are achieved and its targets met, it will see the end to long-stay hospitals and the start of provision of more appropriate accommodation in the community.

The production of a new learning disability development fund of up to £100 million in 2002–2004 is an indication of a financial commitment that has for so long been lacking. It will ensure that the improvements required in the service provision are possible.

National objectives for services for people with a learning disability, supported by new target and performance indicators, bring the service into line with the more mainstream provisions, which are traditionally measured and judged very robustly.

The establishment of a citizen advocacy network and increased funding for self-advocacy organisations in partnership with the voluntary sector will ensure that there is always an independent voice for people with learning disabilities, both as individuals and as a group.

A learning disability award framework is to be established to provide a new qualification route for care workers. This is contentious and there will be ongoing debate about the future needs of formal carers in terms of training and support to carry out the many and various roles they need to adopt.

The success of any service rests both with the people that work within it and the management of the service. It is here where the real challenge lies. It is the coordination of services and the relationships between the wide-ranging service providers and other key stakeholders that will be crucial for the future development of the necessary partnerships and networks. The aim is to give people with a learning disability the opportunity to have as much say and involvement in their lives and related decisions as is possible. It will be imperative that social services, health, education, housing and employment, the benefit agency and others embrace the new philosophy and ensure that the communication problems and barriers of the past are not continued, in order not to hinder progress in the new services. The key challenge is to current staff and managers of organisations to bring about this change. This cannot be achieved without considerable investment in education, training and support.

It is here where we believe that this book will be of value to service providers whatever their background. The style of the chapters is informative and challenging, and the case studies highlight the need to consider the impact of strategy on the lives of the people involved. These case studies are based on real experiences shared by the authors to give invaluable insights into the real world.

There is much to be learnt, in particular from the sensitivity found in the chapters on spirituality, written by Jeanne Males, and bereavement, by Sue Read. These were areas that were largely neglected in the old-style services. This neglect could leave a big deficit in an individual's life, which is being filled today with the new individual and personalised service.

Sexuality and sexual health are also important areas in a person's life. All carers should ensure that they are competent to deal with the issues that people with a learning disability raise with them. If they are not personally competent in this area, they should feel confident to refer on to a specialist therapist or someone with the necessary skills. John Stagg's chapter, which explores the concept of sexuality, is thought provoking as it addresses the issues that matter to an individual. The case studies provided in the chapters by Brian McGinnis, on planning, and Colin Beacock, on mental health and learning disability, offer the reader a perspective and insight not often available to the individual carer or professional.

The recurring theme throughout Lesley Styring's chapter is the acknowledgement that it is good practice to involve people throughout the decision-making process and that much more could be done to overcome the barriers and engage clients and carers in a meaningful way despite the difficulties that face them. This is an interesting and challenging chapter, which will appeal to professionals from all backgrounds. Anne Markwick and Alan Parrish's chapter, 'Older people with learning disabilities', demands that organisations truly face the challenge of engaging individuals in the decision-making process and then are prepared to face the implications of such decisions regardless of the impact on the organisation.

Peter Eldridge tackles the difficult and controversial area of ethics in learning disabilities. This is a philosophical concept rather than a science and will undoubtedly provoke a great deal of debate. We believe that this debate is much needed and perhaps overdue.

Brian Kay nicely draws the book to its conclusion looking at the philosophical issues over the years affecting people with learning disabilities, in two thought-provoking chapters.

A great deal of thought, consideration and effort has gone into the production of this book. Much of the discussion before publication has been prolonged and painful but we believe that this book represents yet another chapter in the evolving story that describes the journey of people with learning disabilities towards their goal of true integration and equality in society.

REFERENCES

Department of Health and Social Security 1971 Better services for the mentally handicapped. HMSO, London

Department of Health 1989 Caring for people. HMSO, London

Department of Health 1992a Health services for people with learning disabilities (mental handicap) (HSG (92) 42). HMSO, London

Department of Health 1992b Social care for adults with learning disabilities (mental handicap) (LAC (92) 15). HMSO, London

Department of Health 2001 Valuing people: a new strategy for learning disability for the 21st century (Cm 5086). The Stationery Office, London

2

Spirituality

Jeanne Males

OVERVIEW
Learning disability presents a particular challenge in terms of definition and terminology, and it is no surprise that to write on 'spirituality' in the context of learning disability is even more of a challenge. It is necessary to begin by addressing something of the meaning of spirituality, giving a few working definitions, and then to go on to discuss which aspects need to be reconsidered in the context of working with individuals with learning disabilities. This chapter does not attempt to make a precise definition of spirituality. An understanding of spirituality is necessarily broad and should not be tied to formal religious practice. It does reflect the ways in which individuals seek to understand their relationships with the things and people around them, and in particular with the things in life that are beyond an immediate understanding.

SPIRITUALITY
The word spirituality is both very frequently used—for it is something in which individuals appear to have a serious and enduring interest—and often misunderstood. Given that the chapter author is a Christian minister, many examples given will inevitably relate to the Christian faith; however, it is hoped that there will be an immediate relevance to the other great world religions and to other spiritual traditions. There are a number of general definitions that are enlightening.

Toon (1989) suggested, in general terms, that 'Spirituality is all about the human search for identity, meaning, purpose, God, self-transcendence, mystical experience, integration and inner harmony. Thus there are spiritualities related to all religions and to many human pursuits which arise in the human spirit.' Leech (1997) commented that it was not surprising that a quest for a deepening spirituality did not often lead to a relationship with the mainstream religions, which were, in his view, marked by 'moderation, compromise and loss of confidence'.

Males and Boswell (1990), in acknowledging the difficulty in defining spirituality, suggested that it concerns the way in which people understand existence, and the actions that proceed from such an understanding. They suggested that spirituality does not involve the acquisition of information or factual knowledge but, 'a reverence for the mysteries of life which no-one can fully understand'. In a similar vein, Murray and Zetner (1989) suggested that spirituality is 'a quality that goes beyond religious affiliation, that strives for reverence, awe, meaning and purpose', and Ipgrave (2001) described a yearning for that which is both beyond us and yet also very close to us. Gillman (2000) helpfully wrote of the role of relationships in his attempt to define spirituality: relationship with the self, the other (neighbour, community) and the environment. He then proceeded to elaborate this as a series of relationships that are infused by the Holy Spirit.

SPIRITUALITY AND LEARNING DISABILITY

These definitions of spirituality—which contain few measurable standards—may at first sight be unhelpful in the context of working in a holistic manner with individuals with a learning disability. It is probably for this reason that, when working with people with learning disability, a consideration of spirituality becomes a box that is ticked either if the individual is regularly taken to a recognised place of worship or if they receive visits or some other kind of support from a chaplain (of whatever faith) who specialises in learning disability. This response can be rightly challenged and replaced with a more creative set of responses.

It may be more useful to begin with Therese Vanier's suggestion, quoted in Linehan (1990), that 'By "spiritual" we mean the need of the whole person to be themselves'. While this is possibly easier to understand, it is also problematic for those who wish for a working definition that will allow for the derivation of working aims and objectives, and measurable standards and outcomes. In addition, whichever working definition might be accepted as being most appropriate, it is clear that a simplistic view of spirituality which leads to an understanding of 'spiritual needs' as being related to attendance at places of worship is at best inappropriate and at worst quite unacceptable.

It is evident that staff will need guidance if they are to contribute to this area of an individual's life. Very recently, Bradford Social Services, Bradford Community Health NHS Trust and Bradford Interfaith Education Centre (2001) have produced guidance for staff working with people with learning disability in their area. The guidance document offers a working definition (p 13) as follows.

The word spiritual has many meanings. Here it can refer to the essence of human beings as unique individuals. 'What makes me, me and you, you?' So it is the power, energy and hopefulness in a person. It is life at its best, growth and creativity, freedom and love. It is what is deepest in us—what gives us direction, motivation. It is what enables a person to survive bad times, to be strong, to overcome difficulties, to become themselves.

These guidance notes, possibly because they emanate from interfaith work, inevitably fall into the trap of being 'religion-focussed' in their interpretation of spiritual needs. Other workers, who also focussed on an organisation-wide approach to improving spiritual care, made a very definite attempt to emphasise the non-religious aspect of spirituality; otherwise, they suggested, it would seem that a non-religious person was not open to spiritual experience (Curtis, Smithers and Golding, 2000).

Historical awareness of spiritual needs in learning disability

These definitions and ways of understanding the essence of spirituality all point to something that is very important to individuals, and possibly very intimate within their lives. This is, indeed, an area that is 'beyond the acquisition of facts' and also beyond traditional measurement and assessment or evaluation. It is, therefore, not surprising that this aspect of life has been largely ignored in the past by those who work with people with learning disability, and this is worth acknowledging in order to understand the influences of history.

Males (1981) argued that the history of care and treatment of people with learning disability has had an inevitable effect on current attitudes. He referred to early views (dating to about the sixteenth century) which, at one extreme, suggested that children with such disabilities were incapable of evil and were themselves angels from heaven, while at the other extreme suggesting that the devil had stolen a human child and substituted himself for it. These early views, whilst inextricably connected with religion, were unlikely to result in any recognition of spirituality in the individual and were more likely, in fact, to create a fear of the person.

The middle to late nineteenth century witnessed the beginnings of the eugenics movement and a suggestion that people who were 'different' were a threat to the continued purity of society (Males, 1981). This led to the segregation of people with learning disability into institutions, and a failure to provide individual and focussed care inevitably arose. The spirituality of a person was hardly an area of concern in this context, as the individuals were not considered worthy of such consideration or respect.

The history that many people with learning disability carry with them is often merely one of 'receiving care' and having things done to them, rather than being helped to grow and develop as an individual personality. Even in the early 1970s when a stronger focus on helping people to learn new skills was evident, personal development and respect for the individual remained largely ignored. The acquisition of skills that could be summed up as 'social competence' very often remained the focus of successful work with an individual, and few other areas received attention.

The philosophy of normalisation (Wolfensberger, 1972) and subsequent work by O'Brien (1981) involved the fundamental premise of valuing each individual and led to the development of the now famous 'Five Service Accomplishments'. These were community presence, competence, choice, status and community participation. Bradford Social Services et al. (2001) argued that these are all ways of promoting spiritual well-being for a person with learning disability.

RECOGNISING AND ASSESSING SPIRITUAL NEEDS The recognition and assessment of spiritual needs are naturally interrelated in a holistic approach to care, which has now rightly gained importance. Curtis, Smithers and Golding (2000) commented that it is impossible to suggest that holistic care is being offered if a person's spirituality is not recognised. It is also acknowledged that spiritual needs are rarely recognised at all, let alone assessed or met within a service provision, even though this must be to neglect the true meaning of a 'holistic' approach to working with people with learning disability.

An assessment of spiritual needs could, however, appear to be a rather unusual concept: many people might say that spirituality is too 'personal' and perhaps too private to be assessed in any way at all. However, unless the area is addressed in some way it will be largely ignored, especially for people who do not either self-advocate or have someone to speak for them. This is the situation for many people with more severe disabilities. Care management often requires that spiritual needs are addressed and it has been the author's experience that it is at this point that a description of attendance at a place of worship, either by the individual or their family, is seen to suffice—and that action to meet any needs is to ensure that such attendance is facilitated. Perhaps a 'worst case' could be that a member of one faith is encouraged to attend the place of worship of another faith, with a justification to the effect that their family 'didn't mind'.

Bradford Social Services et al. (2001) have provided a helpful checklist for staff. It comprises a list of questions for staff to ask themselves about what they have discovered concerning the person with whom they are working. It is suggested that the answers are recorded so that they can be shared by all staff to ensure a consistent approach. The checklist is very useful, but all the questions relate to affiliation to a particular faith—even in relation to diet, use of particular names, personal care and so on. The issue of the way in which an individual relates to their faith is highlighted, but there is little advice as to how a person who has chosen to have little or nothing to do with their faith background might best be helped. Indeed, the document itself set out to be 'interfaith' and focuses mainly on Christianity, Hinduism, Islam, Judaism and Sikhism.

Curtis et al. (2000) have taken a more truly holistic view that will be helpful in thinking more widely about the spiritual well-being of an individual. They have devised an assessment form to be completed as far as is possible with the person with learning disability. It asks questions about whether the person is able to 'demonstrate' what gives them hope, strength, joy and comfort; it looks at positive relationships and whether the person feels loved and/or loves another person. Access to people who are loved and to experiences that give joy or strength is noted. It is only at that stage in the assessment that 'formal' religion is highlighted, for example an understanding of God or gods, ways of worship and attendance at a place of worship. The authors reported that when this assessment tool was piloted it was found to help staff to think more widely about spirituality, and not just about religious practice. Such a means of assisting staff is significant and must be acknowledged: the help that staff and other workers need will be discussed later in the chapter but should always be understood as being essential to any worthwhile contribution. Hoeksema (1995) underlines this issue. This approach to highlighting needs in this area appears to be both creative and very helpful in addressing the needs of individuals, even though it cannot be said to be anything other than a subjective method of assessment.

DISCOVERING SPIRITUALITY IN PEOPLE WITH LEARNING DISABILITY

As with so many aspects of life, things are the same for people with learning disability as they are for people who have not received that label! Consequently, as in the whole of life, much is discovered about a person's spirituality almost accidentally, through observation and through listening. At the same time, it is possible to learn about the spirituality of an individual in a fairly formalised way; a specific attempt can be made to consider the matter, to work in a specific way and to report it. Most importantly, it is necessary to recognise that spiritual needs differ from person to person (Males and Boswell, 1990). Sadler (2001) expresses this most effectively: 'People with learning disabilties are like everyone: unique people with a unique experience of God, of prayer, of life. Generalisations are always limiting.'

Listening

Everyone who works in any capacity with people, particularly those with learning disability, is now aware of the prime importance of *listening* to the people they work with. The advocacy and particularly the self-advocacy movements that began in the 1970s in the USA have had a profound effect on how people with learning disability are understood, and also on service organisation. 'User representation' has become commonplace both in the statutory and voluntary sector, often at all levels in an organisation.

In listening to an individual—and in taking what is said seriously—it is often possible to discover at a deeper level what they are concerned about (Box 2.1). (Examples that relate to the personal experience of the author have had all personal details changed to protect the identitiy of the individual.) Susan could clearly see two types of hurt. The issues may be of very immediate concern indeed, affecting the person in a very real way. For individuals such as Jennifer (Box 2.2), the opportunity to be listened to often for short periods had a profound effect.

Box 2.1	**Susan**
	Susan, a middle aged woman who had lived in a variety of care settings for the whole of her life was asked if anyone had ever hurt her. Her response was a clear 'No'. She went on to say: 'Being hurt means two things. One is when someone hits you, the other is when your boyfriend finishes with you.'

Box 2.2	**Jennifer**
	Jennifer was 31 years old and was dying. She lived in a group home set in a suburban community. She was aware of how ill she was and was beginning to realise that her life would now be very short. As her birthday approached, she said: 'I don't want to die when I'm 32'. Her comment allowed for a brief exploration of how she really felt about her situation. It was only possible to speak for a short time because of the physical and emotional pain she was experiencing at the time. Many brief visits allowed for some acceptance of her situation, as well as expression of her anger. She died at home.

Listening allows the spirituality of the individual to be shared to the benefit of all concerned. This can often occur effectively when people with learning disability live alongside non-disabled people. The L'Arche communities were founded by Jean Vanier in 1964 and are places where people with learning disability and people who have no such label live together in community. L'Arche is rooted in Christian denominations and is ecumenical, but it does accept people of all faiths (or none). Internationally, it is multifaith (there are 117 communities in 31 countries linked through the Federation of L'Arche). Nicholas Ellerker lived in a L'Arche community in South London and is the subject of a short book written by Therese Vanier (1993). The cover note reads: 'Nick Ellerker was no angel. But he was endowed with gifts of the heart. Profoundly human, he had a passion for reconciliation and unity. Helping those around him to live in the present moment, his compassion led him from deep sadness to explosions of joy. And Nick had Down's syndrome … His simple and profound spirituality as well as his rumbustious humanity, live on in these pages to inspire wonder and admiration …' Many people, both disabled and non-disabled, had lived with Nick in community and, above all else, had listened to him. 'Sue … remembers him as having an awareness of the world of political and social issues and of what was happening to others … [she] also remembers a day when the whole household spent the afternoon in the beautiful house and garden of the parents of an assistant. Nick … walked to a vantage point from which there was a lovely view, and began reflecting very perceptively on the difference between this situation and his own background in the suburbs of London.' (p 14, 15) Here it is clear that Nick's spirituality was shared by those who would listen.

Observing   Some people with a learning disability are unable to express them-selves verbally, and it is exactly this group of people—the most severely disabled—who are often omitted when such issues as spirituality are discussed and debated. It may be necessary to *observe* what is happening. Foster (2000) reported from an account of a mother taking her disabled daughter to visit a church near to the daughter's community home. He quotes the mother's account (Dyer, 1996): 'For inexplicable reasons, since the church interior is dark and rather gloomy, Hilary becomes animated there; she laughs, moves her body and makes sounds to replace speech'.

In a different way, it is possible to observe the behaviour of very profoundly disabled people. It is here that people very often agonise about the meaning of the presence of an individual, for the level of response is so small that it is difficult if not impossible to interpret. The observation on Jessica (Box 2.3) should merely stand alone.

Box 2.3	**Jessica**

Jessica was 30 years old. She was a woman who spent her days motionless, unless she was moved by other people—which was regular as staff sought to ensure that her own lack of movement did not cause her additional physical difficulties. Jessica possessed so little ability to respond that she was generally considered to have neither sight nor hearing; more complex assessments had not been carried out because of her fragile state.

She appeared to communicate with no one, and yet it was often said that her silent presence was one of peaceful acceptance that made people re-evaluate their own worries, and the 'crises' they brought with them.

The degree that Jessica felt at ease with her own situation was impossible to assess, and yet she offered a great deal to other people, by silently offering a reappraisal of their own sense of well-being.

Such observations, and perhaps the insights that flow from them, are often born of a long-standing relationship with an individual. It is not easy to 'assess' spiritual needs except within such a relationship, for it is there that an appreciation of such important aspects of an individual will develop and grow. L'Arche communities allow for such insights to grow in a natural way, and the faith context of the life of those communities allows spiritual issues to become very obvious. Nick Ellerker's understanding of ecumenical issues within the Christian faith flowed from such a lifestyle, as graphically described by Therese Vanier (1993).

Expressing spirituality through art

The spirituality of an individual is not only expressed in what they say or how they appear to react to specific circumstances. George Ellis is a well-recognised artist who began his life in institutional care and who now lives in a community home. He has expressed many things about his life through his visual artwork. His disabilities, which are visual and auditory as well as a learning disability, are strongly reflected in his two- and three-dimensional work, which has been much exhibited over a period of over 20 years. He is certainly influenced by the media but is also very strongly affected by the natural world and by the seasons of the year, including the seasons of the church's year. A Nativity scene in three dimensions, created in the1980s largely out of recycled materials, is significant in expressing this last aspect of his work (Surrey Oaklands Art Therapy Collection, 2001). The work of George Ellis was encouraged and nurtured through a department of art therapy.

Expressing spirituality through music and drama

It is equally true that expressions of an individual's spirituality may evolve through music or drama therapy. These means of helping such expression are also reflected in the Creative Arts Retreat Movement, which encourages people to express themselves in new and creative ways in the context of a retreat. In working in this way with a man who suffers from autism and whose communication is severely limited, Sadler (2001) discovered that this man understood a particular Bible story at a very deep level. Sadler advocates the use of drawing, painting and claywork as ways of understanding the spiritual life of severely and profoundly disabled men and women.

Silence

It may be that spirituality is best discovered within the context of silence. This is always difficult to experience, and it is often the case that people with learning disability are thought to be unable to be silent: a common misconception often implies that they are almost incapable of being silent. And yet it is the author's experience that if helped to attain a period of silence—perhaps merely by being asked first to put their books or papers (or bags) in a safe place—they are able to hold silence more effectively than those who are not learning disabled.

Formal religion Formal religious practice will also assist in discovering something about the spirituality of an individual. The days are now long past when everyone was 'required' to attend church, as in the days of institutional care where church attendance was close to an army church parade. People decide to attend a place of religious worship or not, and, in general, denominational boundaries are ignored. Balzikas and O'Hare (1994) described a group home that opened almost opposite a local parish church, and where two men with learning disability decided that they wished to attend church. The way in which that particular faith community accepted and encouraged the two men is a good model. McNair and Smith (2000) noted that there are many practical benefits in addition to meeting spiritual needs that accrue from church attendance; nonetheless, they highlight spiritual needs as the first reason. They reported a small survey of people with learning disability in California, which suggested that 52% of the people surveyed attended church. Even considering the difficulties of a survey with a group of people with learning disability, and the difference in cultural backgrounds, this may be an important marker.

One of the more formal ways in which spiritual issues are discovered and highlighted is within the context of helping people through religious rites of passage. For example, contact may be very important around the time that individuals are preparing for Confirmation or a similarly important step in their faith journey. Rabjohns (1997) wrote simply about supporting a young man through this process and the ways in which she observed his growth. Her brief discussion concerning whether others in the care team thought that this was 'right' is significant in that this attitude may also be reflected in the faith community itself, in the way the church either accepts or fails to accept members who have a learning disability. This was discussed by Bradford (1985) from a theological viewpoint; he suggested a sensitive and integrated Confirmation preparation so that individuals can be supported in attending preparation with other members of a congregation. In practice, the most effective approach is often one that uses both individual preparation and attendance at a group along with other candidates. Personal experience has shown that an additional means of preparation is to facilitate attendance at particular liturgies, such as the Way of the Cross, and to allow the liturgy to 'speak for itself'. This particular devotion is sometimes known as the Stations of the Cross and follows Christ's sufferings from the time he was condemned to death to his death on the cross. It is often used during Lent and Holy Week. Particular points on the journey (often visually illustrated) are a focus for prayer and meditation.

MEETING THE SPIRITUAL NEEDS OF PEOPLE WITH LEARNING DISABILITY
The carer's role

It should go without saying that specific help in meeting spiritual needs should only be given if an individual consents. To identify the 'spiritual' within a person is one important area of work; however, that same person, like many people in our society, may wish to exercise the right not to explore it, not to try to develop that side of their personhood, not to meet those needs. This may be a right that is clearly expressed verbally, but it may also need to be interpreted by others from the individual's behaviour. Sadler (2001) wrote of working as a 'prayer companion' with a woman with multiple disabilities: 'The only sign was that she did not resist coming back the next day, which those who knew her better than I, said was significant'.

To assert that the individual who is learning disabled has a choice does not, in turn, permit such choice to be made by those who are carers. Hoeksema (1995) discussed this matter and suggested that the issue might best be understood in so far as carers should be seen as *supporting* the disabled person in what they wish to do and possibly as *connecting* that person with those who could help, perhaps more naturally, 'such as family members, friends, co-workers, neighbors, *and members of churches and synagogues*' (p 290, italics are original). In the current social climate where freedom of religious expression is protected and upheld at all costs, this is an important issue. It should be clear that to support an individual does not mean that the same beliefs or traditions are upheld; similarly, to take an individual to a place of worship does not mean that the carer is of that same tradition. What is necessary is that the individual is helped to be at a place of worship (for example) and given any practical help they need in order to participate in the worship. This may mean taking an individual to receive Holy Communion when this is little understood by the carer (or indeed where its very meaning is rejected by the carer). This may be difficult and challenging but is a necessary part of meeting *all* the spiritual needs of an individual. Foster (2000) made the following comment in this vein: 'A learning disabled friend of mine was recently unable to attend church one Sunday morning because a newly appointed carer would not take him, the carer claiming that "he did not believe that sort of thing". Like many others, I find this appalling and would want to ask the carer if he would refuse to take the client to a concert because he did not like the music being played? Professional carers have a clear responsibility to provide for clients' needs on a holistic basis, irrespective of the carers' own beliefs and value systems.'

The nature of support required

Having established the professional responsibility to help, the nature of help given needs to be identified. Carers may themselves require support in this type of service provision, as may others involved in meeting spiritual needs. Christian ministers of religion, for example, are known to be often lacking in education about disability and are consequently anxious about how to help people who are learning disabled within their faith communities.

A fundamental point is that it is necessary to help to meet spiritual needs in as many ways as possible, and using all the senses. In understanding traditional forms of worship, it is usually helpful to begin from an understanding that people can use all their senses in worship. This is particularly important when working with people who have profound and often multiple disabilities, where it is vital that help is given using the most appropriate senses to meet specific needs. This point is made in a short published interview that looked at ways in which the church can help (Parrish, Boswell and Males, 1988). It described a church introducing the use of incense because it was served by two people who had no hearing or speech. Sadler (2001) suggested that a variety of different methods should be used in helping people to express themselves, especially with people with more complex disabilities. The author's experience in running a Quiet Day for people with learning disability has been that as great a variety of approaches as possible should be used: singing, dance, drama, story telling, quietness and individual work, including walking in the countryside. All these activities contributed to a successful Quiet Day where people with disabilities shared with non-disabled people and worked with a non-disabled partner for the day. This approach, along with others in a similar vein, makes some progress towards addressing Edwards (1995), who challenged the full life of the church if it continued to exclude people with learning disability.

L'Arche communities, which were discussed above, do much to help the spiritual life of their members. The Charter of L'Arche is as follows: 'L'Arche communities are places of hope. Each person, according to his or her own vocation, is encouraged to grow in love, self-giving and wholeness, as well as in independence, competence and the ability to make choices.' In the UK, the life of L'Arche communities follows the calendar of the church's year, and the exploration and development of the spiritual needs of an individual are fundamental to the life of the community. Regular opportunities for prayer, for exploration of the faith, for retreat and pilgrimage are significant aspects of life.

CONCLUSION Spirituality is difficult to define and covers aspects that involve both formal religion and wider issues such as the need to be oneself and to relate to others. It also involves the person with a learning disability, the carer and the wider community, for example when carers need to facilitate a relationship that goes against their own personal religion or beliefs. It is also important to use all the senses to discover spirituality in those with a learning disability and to enable them to express this. Music, art, drama and organised religion all offer outlets for spirituality by helping communication.

REFERENCES

Balzikas D, O'Hare M 1994 The helping hand of God. Nursing Standard 9(9): 46–47

Bradford J 1985 Preparing the mentally handicapped for confirmation. The Children's Society, London

Bradford Social Services, Bradford Community Health NHS Trust, and Bradford Interfaith Education Centre 2001 Spiritual well-being: policy and practice. Bradford Metropolitan District Council, Bradford

Curtis M, Smithers L, Golding C 2000 The ghost in the machine. Learning Disability Practice 3(2): 11–12

Dyer, B (1996) Seeming Parted, New Millenium, London

Edwards J 1995 Retreats for people with learning disability—why not? St Joseph's Newsletter 51: 2

Foster M 2000 High spirits. Learning Disability Practice 2(4): 16–19

Gillman H 2000 Circles and spirals—some thoughts on the meaning of spirituality. SPIDIR Newsletter 51: 1–2

Hoeksema T B 1995 Supporting the free exercise of religion in the group home context. Mental Retardation 33(5): 289–294

Ipgrave M 2001 Inter-faith spirituality retreats. The Retreat Association, London

Leech K 1997 The sky is red. Darton, Longman and Todd, London

Linehan T 1990 Freeing altar egos. Care Weekly, August 24: 17

Males B 1981 Public attitudes to mental handicap as reflected in the opinion of school children. MA Thesis, University of Keele, UK

Males J, Boswell C 1990 Spiritual needs of people with a mental handicap. Nursing Standard 4(48): 35–37

McNair J, Smith H K 2000 Church attendance of adults with developmental disabilities. Education and Training in Mental Retardation and Developmental Disabilities 35(2): 222–225

Murray R B, Zetner J P 1989 Nursing concepts for health promotion. Prentice Hall, London

O'Brien J 1981 The principle of normalisation: a foundation for effective services. Campaign for Mentally Handicapped People, London

Parrish A, Boswell C, Males J 1988 Spiritual and practical help from the church. Community Living 2(1): 8–9

Rabjohns G 1997 Circle of support. LLAIS 43: 19

Sadler C 2001 Accompanying people with learning disabilities. In: Retreats 2001. The Retreat Association, London, pp 6–7

Surrey Oaklands Art Therapy Collection 2001 George Ellis. Surrey Oaklands Art Therapy, Oaklands, UK

Toon P 1989 What is spirituality? And is it for me? Daybreak, London, pp 14, 15

Vanier T 1993 Nick: man of the heart. Gill and Macmillan, Dublin

Wolfensberger W 1972 The principle of normalisation in human services. National Institute on Mental Retardation, Toronto, Canada

SOURCES

Creative Arts Retreat Movement, 182 High St, Street, Somerset BA16 0AH, UK

L'Arche UK Secretariat, 10 Briggate, Silsden, Keighly, West Yorkshire BD20 9JT, UK

3

Sexuality and people with learning disability

John Stagg

OVERVIEW   This chapter will explore aspects of sexuality in various settings, particularly issues related to working with young people with learning difficulties, and sexual health promotion, including education and risk management. There will also be some consideration of ethical and legal perspectives related to supporting people with learning disabilities and their sexuality needs.

The author has drawn upon his own experiences of working as a nurse for people with learning disabilities in a mainly community setting. Some of the key factors explored will include working with other professionals, formal carers and informal carers. The chapter provides information and exploration of work that others may draw on to build upon their own efforts in supporting people with learning disabilities in an area that is often controversial, always sensitive and frequently difficult.

This chapter discusses the use of assessment programmes that consider lifestyle, networks and past experiences. Discussion of support, using case examples, will show how an understanding of a person's history can assist in identifying that individual's needs.

DEFINING   During a recent multiprofessional supervision session, the author and
SEXUALITY   his colleagues attempted to define sexuality and to discuss how it influenced the group work they were undertaking. After discussion, debate and argument, it was clear that each individual had different concepts, boundaries and ideas about how sexuality could be defined. Some common themes included gender, sexual orientation, age, self-expression and biology. Life experiences and learning were also common to how people defined sexuality.

A useful definition is offered within the discussion and guidance document on sexuality and sexual health in nursing practice produced by the Royal College of Nursing (2000):

> **Sexuality**—an individual's self concept, shaped by their personality and expressed as sexual feelings, attitudes, beliefs and behaviours,

expressed through a heterosexual, homosexual, bisexual or transsexual orientation.

The Royal College of Nursing goes on to offer the following statement concerning sexual health.

> ...the physical, emotional, psychological, social and cultural well being of a person's sexual identity, and the capacity and freedom to enjoy and express sexuality without exploitation, oppression, physical or emotional harm. Sexual health may either be a primary or secondary focus of nursing care, depending on the patient's care needs. This is more apparent for some people who may need specific nursing care to develop and promote sexual health.

Although the above is from a document targeted at nurses, the definition is a useful means of considering sexual health as an issue for people beyond merely the sexual act or sexual problem/need. The reference to patients and nursing care would apply to people with learning disability who require more specific support.

SEXUALITY IN CONTEXT

Sexuality is an integral part of our being: 'To be a human is to be a sexual being' (Craft, 1987). Our expression of our sexuality, our gender, our sexual orientation, sexual likes/dislikes, sexual health and lifestyle are wrapped in sexuality. Although each of us is a unique individual, no one person is any different in the important role sexuality plays in his or her life. Drury et al. (2000) noted that sexuality 'refers to the whole person': not only how our body works but how we think, feel, what we believe and our behaviours towards ourselves and others.

Some aspects of sexuality are inherent or genetic, while others are learned or influenced. This ever-developing and changing facet of ourselves continues to be influenced by ageing and both simple and complex life experiences, positive and negative (Rutter, 2000; Schwier and Hingsburger, 2000).

As we grow and progress through education, we begin to learn more about societal rules and laws, including respecting other people and, hopefully, respecting ourselves. Sexuality is, in turn, integrated with our communication, self-expression, relationships, goals and life events. Much of this we take for granted, or at least without giving our sexuality a great deal of thought except, perhaps, when we become sexually aware and begin to experience attraction and physical changes.

In the majority of people with learning disabilities the author has encountered, there have been other influences affecting this development of sexuality. Some of the influences include changed health (ill-health) or condition; lesser expectations of achievement by others, including 'economic and social marginalisation'; 'dependency'; 'segregation and social exclusion' (Cambridge and McCarthy, 1997); behaviours that challenge; fear; infantalisation; reduced or absent opportunities; vulnerability; and abuse. All influences vary as much as they do for any one person and could not be associated with every individual. Each individual is part of society, influenced by society's norms and expectations. These, in turn, influence the views and attitudes of carers and others involved in the life of the person with a learning disability, a concept discussed by Cooper and Guillebaud (1999).

When one thinks of an example of need and then the likely support or intervention, sexuality will be an integral part of meeting that need, to a greater or lesser extent. Examples of needs might include:

- support for incontinence
- independent living skills
- work
- communication
- social communication difficulties
- personal care needs
- living arrangements and accommodation
- carer support
- bereavement
- financial support or limitations.

It may be a simple aspect of support, such as a carer or friend being of the same age, gender and culture, to allow the individual to feel comfortable with the support being offered. Perhaps dominant role models have been mainly men or women. Personal care and support might be offered in such a way that it unintentionally infantilises the individual. Use of language that pertains to a younger person may describe care in a way which is devaluing. The gender of those living in shared accommodation may present risks.

INCLUSION OF SEXUALITY IN A CARE PLAN

Those with both physical and learning disabilities require support on many levels. The building of an overall care plan and its extension to include aspects of sexuality are illustrated with the needs of a young man, John Spence (Box 3.1).

| Box 3.1 | **John Spence** |

John was admitted to a National Health Service (NHS) residential home at the age of 23. He had been admitted to a long-stay hospital for people with learning disability at around 7 years of age.

John had a severe learning disability as a result of marked cerebral palsy. He was dependent upon his carers to meet all of his needs. He had epilepsy and experienced frequent tonic–clonic seizures and absences and status epilepticus.

John required his carers to carry out all aspects of physical care. He was unable to eat independently, was doubly incontinent and required regular administration of enemas. He could only move around in a wheelchair. John spent much of his day asleep, and when he was awake he would often shout or scream.

John's mother usually visited monthly, his father having died several years earlier. He had two brothers and one sister, none of whom had visited in the last 10 years.

When John arrived at the house, his light brown hair hung down over his face covering his eyes. His crown and the back of his head were bald from constant movement of his head, rubbing on the back of his wheelchair seat. His face was covered in spots. A rash, caused by constant dribbling of saliva, extended from his lower chin to his chest. He wore a pair of shrunk and faded tracksuit bottoms; his jumper was stained with food and was baggy and washed out of shape. There was a strong odour of stale urine and faeces. Beside him were two bin liners containing his possessions. One contained faded damaged clothes and the other a child's activity centre, a broken tape player and several nursery rhyme tapes.

The escorting nurse described him as 'a real baby…who likes to get his own way'. Before leaving she handed over his medication, a short care plan (describing the most basic of care needs) and the details of his finances. A rub on John's cheek, 'Be a good boy,…love him', were her parting words and gestures.

At this point, John was completely unknown. A read through of his care plan and some brief notes gave little information as to who he was. Information was not readily available; his rapid transfer from the hospital was hurried and poorly organised; it had not allowed time for staff to meet John or build any kind of relationship.

His mother Doreen arrived. Doreen was used to a model of care that focused on ill-health. Doreen did reveal that she felt guilty and embarrassed at John's appearance. She admitted that she had long given up trying to provide clothes or possessions that he might like, finding them damaged or missing the next time she visited. She had actively encouraged her other children to break off their contact and pursue their own lives, feeling that John was lost to her and her family. She cared deeply about him but found herself disempowered by services and unable to participate in his care. Eventually, she had broken away, making monthly visits out of a sense of duty while constantly building her feelings of grief and helplessness.

Doreen reluctantly agreed to remain for a meal, staying until John went to bed. She spent time talking about John's past, her husband and her other children. Her information about John, his family and her perception of his needs were invaluable. Perhaps more importantly, she began to rebuild her relationship with her son.

A basic care plan   John had many needs and perhaps the immediate priority was his physical health care. A multidisciplinary care plan was devised that included the following areas:

- A consultant psychiatrist, the nursing staff and the general practitioner (GP) were involved in the assessment, treatment and management of his epilepsy, constipation and skin conditions. His sight and hearing were also assessed, as were his dental needs.

- A physiotherapist devised a treatment programme to reduce contractures and to prevent further deterioration in relation to spasticity. She also reviewed his posture and guided staff in how to move and handle John safely.
- A speech and language therapist advised on eating and communication, which included developing John's care to incorporate total communication within his care.
- A care plan gave detailed information about how to provide personal care, related to washing, bathing and continence, involving two people, at least one of whom was also a man whenever possible. The routine of personal care was provided using a consistent approach, incorporating a free-standing mirror to allow John to be able to see what was happening to him. John had not had the opportunity to see what happened to his body because of his posture and positioning during personal care. Staff would tell John what they were doing, making no assumptions about his understanding of what was being said to him.

Activities, both at home and within the community, were facilitated with a view to building up regular patterns of events to help John to develop awareness and interests. This included providing John with new clothes, possessions and activities.

A comprehensive risk assessment was undertaken relating to management of seizures, moving and handling, stress created by changes in environment and John's vulnerability.

Several months after his move, John rarely slept during the day. His epilepsy was better controlled and his need for regular administration of enemas also reduced. His physical appearance improved, with better attention to his personal and oral hygiene. The bald patches on his head reduced to a small area at the back of his head. His wheelchair seating was reviewed and adapted to give better posture and a safer eating position. John only occasionally became distressed; this was nearly always alleviated through a change of activity, environment, position, or the offer of something to eat or drink.

John also began to initiate contact with people by knocking them with his arm if they went past. It became second nature to respond to John, just as staff would with any other person who was trying to attract their attention. Changes in John's position and in his activities were tried in order to help him to have choices. Other choices were created, for example simply allowing John to taste two types of food or drink and judging his response. Gradually John indicated some preferences related to touch, taste, sound and environment.

If John was positioned appropriately and given food that did not require cutlery to eat, he was able to eat with greater independence. Through trial and error, it became apparent that John had an eclectic taste in music, with specific dislikes of certain sounds and music styles.

John began to build relationships with people in his local community: staff in a local newsagents and his local barber for example. John would respond by looking at people when they said his name and often smiled or laughed. He gradually developed anonymity within busy environments, such as the local supermarket. John's clothes, scent and style became representative of any other man of his age. His physical disability and use of a wheelchair was still an obvious factor, although care was taken not to accentuate these in any way that created a devaluing image.

Integration of sexuality in the basic care plan

The sexual aspects of John's behaviour (Box 3.2) initiated a reassessment of how John's sexuality was acknowledged in the initial care plan and what changes could and should be made as he became better known. The home manager and John's key worker considered his care plan and reviewed John's needs at this point and at the time when he came to live in the house. It became apparent that, in meeting John's needs, staff had integrated many aspects of care. Sexuality had been considered specifically in terms of John's outward appearance and physical care, including the gender of carers. The manager and key worker also considered other elements of support and care that influenced John's expression of sexuality.

Box 3.2	**John Spence cont.**

It became evident that when John was undressed, for example following a bath, he would touch his genitalia, especially his penis. If left to do this, John would attain an erection and derived pleasure from doing this. Initially this was a difficult issue for staff to address because of their feelings of embarrassment and a sense of not knowing what to do.

- His possessions and personal environment reflected those of any other average man of John's age.
- Language used to describe John and his activities, and when communicating with John, was also orientated to John's age and gender. Appropriate terms of reference that reflected positive attitudes and values were routine. For example, terms such as 'feeding' were not evident; instead 'eating' or 'support with eating' were used.
- John's health and his ability to participate in meaningful, facilitated community activity had also been improved.
- John gained experience of other forms of physical touch through sensory work and massage of hands, which gave an alternative experience to only being touched during physical care.

- John was given the opportunity to see what was happening to his body during personal care.

Developing a care plan to include sexuality

There was debate among the staff as to how masturbation should be addressed. Two possibilities were suggested, both with disadvantages:

1. John could be left to carry out his sexual activity alone in his room, lying on his bed. But how would his safety be maintained and how would staff know when to re-enter the room, without being obtrusive or disregarding his need for privacy and space?
2. John could be left to pursue this activity during the time it took to get him dried and dressed following a bath. However, that would significantly reduce any time John had to carry out this activity and may actually prevent it from occurring at all.

Some members of staff were not comfortable to address this issue at all and others felt that it was almost devaluing John to have other people discuss his needs in this way. He could not be included in this type of dialogue and a wider discussion would further breach his privacy.

Ethical issues arising from the care plan

In order to address the issue of masturbation, the manager opted to hold a staff meeting to consider the ethical issues of John's care. Discussion considered both masturbation and other choices in John's life.

Because of the nature of John's learning disability and his limited communication skills, it was impossible to judge whether John could comprehend and retain the relevant information to be able to make a decision and thus have the capacity to consent. Therefore, it was also not possible to know whether John could understand the information given to him, by any means, and decide on aspects of care or other issues. In other words, John was not 'capable of understanding what was proposed and its implications or able to exercise choice' (Letts, 1994).

It was accepted that John could develop some choices, albeit simple ones, which should be viewed as his choices because of positive changes in his behaviour.

A multidisciplinary review was held that involved significant key staff involved with John's care and included the psychiatrist, psychologist and speech and language therapist. The framework used to help with decision making used the ethical problem-solving topics taken from Seedhouse (1988).

To help to frame their discussion, John's needs and how they were being met were mapped out (Fig. 3.1). This helped people to visualise how John's life had developed since coming to live in the house. It also added in new issues or dilemmas that the care team would require to

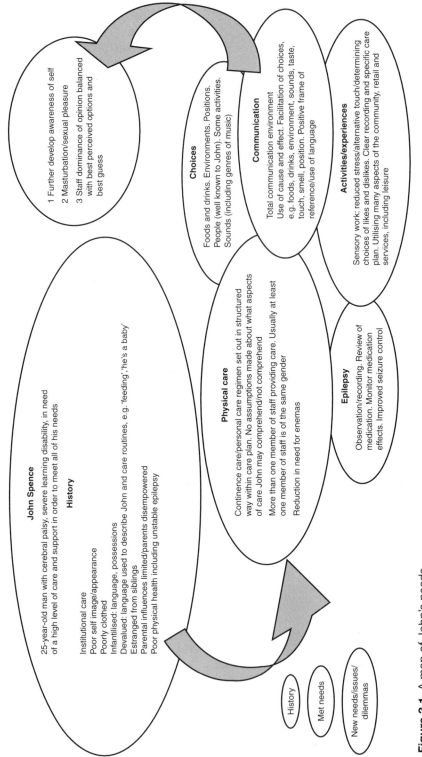

Figure 3.1 A map of John's needs

address. Doreen Spence was not invited to this meeting, the decision made on the basis that Doreen could not consent for John and it was thought unlikely that an adult man would wish to have the intimate need of masturbation/sexual pleasure discussed with his mother. The manager and the key worker decided to have a planning meeting that included discussing the issue of sexual pleasure and then to hold the regular review with Doreen present, which did not include intimate issues of sexual need.

Topics from Seedhouse (1988) were utilised to facilitate discussion.

Wishes of others. This included the ideas and needs of the staff as well as what John's needs and wishes might be if he was able to express these for himself.

Legal rights of both John and staff. Staff should not be asked to carry out any elements of care that breached either John's legal rights or the legal rights of the staff.

The responsibility to justify all actions in terms of external evidence. Any decisions made about John's care and support needed to be justified from a multidisciplinary perspective, which took account of all known factors affecting John, including his past.

Disputed facts and the degree of certainty of evidence on which action is taken. It was essential to debate openly and honestly whether any proposed aspects of care were such that some staff/other professionals could not agree. At the same time, it was necessary to feel sure that any decisions about care were agreed and that the reasons for making decisions were sound.

The risk. Any risk factors affecting psychosocial needs, environment and physical self must be taken into account.

Effectiveness and efficacy of actions. This involved examining current support and ensuring that decisions made about future support were actually meeting John's needs. Again this included devising some means of evaluating care (the outcomes of interventions and actions by staff to support John).

Increase of good. This would be considered in terms of increase of self-good (as opposed to creating harm). It could also apply to issues such as staff influences, wishes or ideas.

Minimise harm. Apart from identifying any immediate risk, there was a need to ensure continuous evaluation to identify whether any potential risks were not being considered and to continue to ensure safe holistic care.

Respect persons equally, create autonomy, respect autonomy. This area would involve ensuring that no aspects of John's needs were not considered on the grounds that he had a learning disability. There was a need to ensure that no one was complacent in continuing to strive to create autonomy and independence for John in any way possible and to maintain existing independence or autonomy.

Serve needs before wants. It was felt that there can be a common theme, in care settings, to avoid giving consideration to sensitive, unpleasant or difficult aspects of practice/care, where there can be difficulty in reaching agreement because of different beliefs, values and ideology.

A modified care and support plan

The care team considered all aspects of care and opted that, in order to continue to promote autonomy, John would be left in his room in a comfortable position on his bed whenever there was any indication that he was becoming sexually aroused. An addendum was made to his care plan to include details of how to allow John to be left on his bed, unsupervised, without the risk of him falling. His nails were to be kept short also. In order to ensure that John was not going to injure himself, staff would make discreet observations of his genitalia afterwards to ensure that he had not caused himself any injury. He had been noted to concentrate his touching to his penis, and this was felt to reduce the risk of him inadvertently injuring his scrotum or testicles. During the initial phase of facilitation, John's key worker and the home manager were to make discreet observations outside John's door, listening for changes in the vocal sounds John might make (i.e. sounds of any distress) including any indication that John had finished masturbating. This helped to ensure that risks were being minimised and gave an approximation of how much time John required without leaving him alone unsupported for too long.

The times when John became sexually aroused tended to follow him having a bath. John was bathed daily and required to be left lying on his bed for 30 minutes. At the end of this time, staff would listen at the door before entering, to ensure that they were not entering inappropriately. Little or no noise indicated that John was not masturbating. Staff would then resume caring for John, carrying out any personal care that was required.

It was also agreed that this process would be reviewed, initially on a weekly basis. Confidential notes were kept in order that changes in the times John became aroused could be considered as well as how long John required to be left alone.

Discussion ensued as to the views and feelings of the staff. One member of staff felt that encouraging masturbation might infringe on religious beliefs. Doreen had disclosed that John's family religion had not been observed since John's christening. He had never been brought up observing many practices, other than those that were additionally signified by holidays. To introduce a particular belief, practice or concept would be generated by another person's philosophy, which John would not be able to internalise for himself.

It was felt that if John had not needed to use incontinence products, he would have had the freedom to touch his genitalia when undressed or when he was wearing limited clothing, for example during the night. The plan was a staff response to one of John's behaviours rather than an attempt to facilitate something that did not already exist. Whether or not John had 'capacity' to consent in general terms, it was clear that he was feeling sexually aroused and staff were attempting to respond to this complex need (Aylott, 1999). Staff were not applying their own values or beliefs in deliberately encouraging a behaviour (sexual arousal) but were responding to arousal that occurred naturally. In addition, the initial steps to evaluate the approach taken would allow for appropriate adaptation, which could include discontinuing this support. Continuous monitoring of John's care plan ensured that needs were met in a safe way.

The quote from the late Ann Craft (1987) has been used in texts before and perhaps encapsulates, better than most statements, what carers might consider when supporting people with learning disability in relation to sexuality.

> To be a human being is to be a sexual being. Although there may be a range of intensity, varying over time, we all have sexual needs, feelings and drives, from the most profoundly handicapped to the most able among us. Although we can shape (and mis-shape) sexual expression, sexuality is not an optional extra which we in our wisdom can choose to bestow or withhold according to whether or not some kind of intelligence test is passed.

SEXUAL CARE SUPPORT IN A SEMI-SUPPORTED SETTING

Many individuals with learning disabilities lead semi-independent lives and will encounter many of the problems of sexuality seen by all in society. They may be less able to realise their needs or know who to go to for support; they will, therefore, have particular needs. These needs may not be the immediately apparent ones, such as contraceptive advice, and assessment becomes an important feature of delivering the correct support. The provision and development of care support for a young person regarding a relationship is illustrated with Jane Martin, a 24-year-old woman with a learning disability who lived in a semi-supported scheme (Box 3.3).

Box 3.3	Jane Martin

Jane was a 24-year-old woman living in a semi-supported housing scheme. Each house had up to four occupants; women and men shared each house, with all house mates having their own bedroom and sharing other communal areas. Staff supported clients, individually or as a group, with skills development, organisation and general problem solving. Most people utilised one day per week when they remained in their home to carry out their own chores, shopping and to gain support with independent living skills.

Jane had recently developed a relationship with a man, Thomas, who lived in one of the other homes run by the service. He was a frequent visitor to Jane's house, being particularly friendly with two of Jane's house mates.

Jane was referred by her key worker Maggie to the local Community Learning Disability Team for support and advice in gaining contraception.

Jane was referred by her key worker Maggie to the local Community Learning Disability Team (CLDT). The referral requested 'some advice and protection now that Jane is exploring her sexuality'. Maggie explained to the visiting nurse Alan that Jane required contraception as a result of her relationship with Thomas.

Jane was quiet during the meeting and it became apparent that Maggie was answering questions for Jane or prompting her with leading questions. Jane had not understood why she was being referred and had not agreed to the referral, or the meeting. It became apparent that Jane was not clear that she wanted to have any kind of contraception either.

Confidentiality It is important to establish with clients and carers ground rules related to confidentiality. This ensures that people are aware of their rights to privacy and encourages appropriate expectations of others. It also reduces the risk of the service user feeling let down or betrayed, and it avoids the worker being in a vulnerable position of having to break confidence when faced with a dilemma involving serious risk/harm to the person they are supporting. It is useful to write these ground rules down and/or devise some kind of visual contract as a reminder. This confidentiality contract can then be revisited to remind people of what has been agreed. Sometimes this requires to be done at each meeting.

Alan explained to Jane, in non-euphemistic language, the ground rules related to confidentiality, stating that whatever was discussed was between Jane and Alan. Alan would only discuss issues with someone else if he felt that there were any risks or harm to Jane involved. He would tell Jane about these and who he would need to tell. Alan took some time to work through this with Jane, encouraging her to reflect her understanding of what he had said, until he felt that Jane had understood these confidentiality issues. At this stage Maggie left the room, with the option that she could return at any time Jane wished her to do so.

Defining needs   Jane gradually relaxed and was able to discuss the referral. Jane had developed a relationship with Thomas, but it was unclear from Jane's description that it was anything more than a friendship. Alan established that Jane did not understand what contraception was about and had difficulty expressing concepts of relationships. Alan felt that assessment would be helpful to establish the following:

- Jane's communication skills/needs
- Jane's sexual knowledge
- Jane's comprehension and ways in which she understood information.

Assessment information would help to pitch any intervention appropriately so that it was accessible to Jane and of help in establishing her capacity to consent to issues within a sexual relationship, if indeed this was an issue. (There is no defined tool to make a test of capacity in law. However, the common law test of capacity must show that the person be capable of understanding what is proposed and its implications and that the person must be able to exercise choice.)

Alan discussed these ideas with Jane, explaining how they may be helpful. Alan also suggested that Maggie would perhaps be able to provide support if Jane wanted this. Jane was keen that Maggie should be involved and agreed to meet other people from the team, namely a speech and language therapist and a psychologist. Alan also suggested that he and Jane meet the domiciliary family planning nurse, Kathy, who might offer Jane some support in the future, especially regarding sexual health screening.

At the end of this preliminary discussion, several useful strands of information had been elicited. The first was Jane's needs. Alan finished the meeting by describing what he felt Jane's needs might be. Alan and Maggie agreed to carry out a risk assessment together to ensure that Jane was not at risk and that her needs were being met. The second issue was Thomas, who was also in need of support. He was possibly more able than Jane but would not have insight into her needs. The third issue was how the support staff had viewed and dealt with Jane's situation. Maggie realised that she and her colleagues had not considered Jane's ability in such depth, concerned that they were not infringing her privacy while trying to maintain her ability to access appropriate health services. Maggie was able to consider how future staff training might address these issues.

Assessment   Assessments revealed that Jane presented as a fairly able woman with good language skills; this disguised some deficits of ability in terms of memory and being able to retain information. Jane often gave the impression of understanding what was said to her although explorative questioning revealed that she only partially understood information. The use of complex language was difficult for Jane and she required to be given short pieces of information. It assisted Jane to understand and remember information if cues and reminders were visual, perhaps using line drawings or pictures.

Jane also had difficulty in sequencing some tasks; this was disguised by people prompting her into the next stage of an activity, although frequently repeated activities or those that utilised visual cues did not present a problem. Jane also had many practical skills at which she was competent. She was able to care for herself without any prompting or support and made appropriate choices about her appearance. Jane could manage with expected issues, such as catching a bus at a particular place and time. She could also cope well with money, as long as she was adequately prepared beforehand: that is, if she used a list and knew what the likely costs would be. Jane did not read well, but she was able to recognise familiar words or objects; therefore, she could cope with purchasing familiar items unless the packaging changed. Jane could predict some aspects of consequence of an action or situation fairly well, although her prediction of social situations was fairly poor. Assessment demonstrated that Jane could have poor skills in relation to self-protection if she overly trusted people and she had no healthy suspicion of their intentions.

Jane also had deficits in being able to recognise some aspects of emotion. Using 'emotion picture cards' to assess Jane's interpretations of feelings, it became apparent that she confused feeling 'tired' with feeling 'sad' and feeling 'angry' with feeling 'excited'.

Jane had been employed part time in an animal sanctuary for 3 years, which she enjoyed. She had positive relationships with work colleagues but did not tend to socialise with them. At home, Jane enjoyed watching television and carried out some social activities with the people she lived with and other friends. Jane had been involved in two other relationships with men, who she described as boyfriends.

Additional assessment Alan met Jane to carry out the Sexual Knowledge Assessment from the Brooks Advisory Centre (1987), which he adapted by including additional pictorial information from other teaching resources, namely *You me and HIV* (O'Sullivan and Gillies, 1993), *Picture yourself* (Dixon, 2002) and *Sex and the 3Rs* (McCarthy and Thompson, 1992). This provided a baseline assessment of knowledge of the body, relationships, intercourse, conception, contraception, pregnancy, giving birth, parenting (basic awareness) and abuse. This helped to identify specific areas of learning need in relation to:

- sexual intercourse
- self-protection (avoiding abuse)

- pregnancy
- conception and contraception.

Jane had some knowledge of these issues but had misconceptions or poor awareness, which made her vulnerable to being abused. Through the assessment, it became known that Thomas was carrying out contact abuse: trying to touch Jane, which she did not wish to happen. Contact abuse is identified by Brown and Turk (1992) as touching the body, genitalia and breasts, and that this contact may also involve unwanted intercourse, vaginal or anal, and oral sex. Thomas had made several attempts to touch Jane's body, both her breasts and upper thighs. It was important at this point to stop further discussion and, using the confidentiality ground rules, Alan was able to explain to Jane that they both needed to talk to Jane's social worker and to Maggie. Jane's social worker made a visit to discuss with Jane her disclosure of abuse. (Abuse is explored within a separate chapter of this book and has, therefore, not been discussed further.)

Further support Jane also met with the family planning nurse Sally, who had worked with professionals within the CLDT and had developed a networking arrangement with the team. Sally, Alan and Jane met on several occasions, which allowed Jane gradually to understand Sally's role and what kind of support she offered. Jane was also able to describe to Sally the work she had undertaken with Alan. Sally also sat in on two of the sessions.

Alan utilised information from the teaching packs listed earlier and included slides from *Life horizons I* and *II* (Kempton, 1988). These teaching resources provided Jane with visual information to help with her understanding and development of knowledge. The addition of the slides within the *Life horizons* packs provided 'life' pictures. Sally utilised some of this material to help Jane to gain a better understanding of sexual health needs, such as breast awareness and cervical screening. Knowledge of menstruation (periods), including monitoring and coping with periods, and self-care were also included as aspects of support.

Sally was able to move to having individual sessions with Jane and explore other aspects of sexual enjoyment. Jane was able to talk about her masturbation technique and realised that, although she had felt guilty about this, she was not causing herself any harm and that it was a natural and pleasurable activity.

Following a series of combined teaching sessions with Alan and Sally, Jane developed a greater knowledge of her own body, her sexual life cycle, love making, partnerships and sexual health; she also developed a greater ability to be assertive. Jane did not want to have a sexual partner and did not want to accept contraception. After 36 weekly sessions, the Sexual Knowledge Assessment was repeated, which demonstrated an overall improvement in basic knowledge especially of situations that were abusive rather than potentially abusive. Jane still had some areas of need, in predicting some outcomes or preventing abusive situations occurring. This remained a need that services required to consider when providing future support.

A final care plan

There were three aspects to the conclusions of Jane's assessment. With regard to Jane herself, her disclosure of contact abuse resulted in her receiving additional supportive counselling, which occurred concurrently with the educational and sexual health support. Counselling was provided by a psychosexual counsellor who worked in partnership with the CLDT. The counsellor was guided by the information gained from the assessments undertaken by members of the team, which informed her approach in supporting Jane.

Thomas also began to receive support, initially on an individual basis and later he attended a men's group that focussed on social communication skills, including roles, rights and responsibilities.

Finally, there was a shift in culture within the residential service, which accepted that greater care may be required in actually facilitating developing relationships. Care was required to ensure that service users were able to access other support agencies in terms of sexual health, sexual needs and relationships. In their attempt to support Jane, staff may have unwittingly allowed abuse to have been perpetrated. Had staff not taken steps to protect Jane, or had they disregarded the information and decisions made by Jane and her social worker, then the agency may have been liable under the Sexual Offences Act 1956, which states that it is an offence for 'A person who is the owner or occupier of any premises, or has, or acts or assists in, the management or control of any premises, to induce or knowingly suffer a woman who is a defective to resort to or be on those premises for the purpose of having unlawful sexual intercourse with men or a particular man'. The law relating to sexual offences is currently under review and, although unlikely to change, the proposed definition of capacity to consent will be based on that proposed by the Law Commission (2000). This contains a series of proposed recommendations that, as and when adopted as part of the legislative, must be considered when supporting people with learning disabilities in aspects of sexuality and sexual health.

A SEX EDUCATION GROUP

Most young people attend sex education within their school setting; this, for most, is a repeated and ongoing event. There is usually an emphasis on biological functions rather than social and relationship skills. This common factor is discussed by Fegan, Rauch and McCarthy (1993), who considered that this can be an inappropriate focus. Once young people move beyond secondary education they are often without support and often in need of it. The following section discusses the formation of a sex education group for young people with learning disabilities who were students at a college of further education. The students were aged between 18 and 20 years and attended the college full time.

Course design The course was designed to last for 2 years and the overall aim was to extend the individual's education and engender practical skills leading to employment and/or further training. An ongoing theme of developing social skills was evident throughout the course.

A meeting with the course leaders and the author was arranged to discuss the overall content and consider what support could be offered.

The course leaders wanted to work in partnership to develop sessions that would meet needs. Social skills development was already incorporated into what the students would be undertaking generally. There were no plans to provide any specific support. One of the tutors, a woman, was to co-facilitate the group and help to support the women with specific issues. More detailed or complex support would be discussed by the facilitators, with the option of supporting the student to refer on for specific professional advice.

A review took place of the intended format and several factors were identified. The following questions were raised:

1. What was going to be achieved?
2. How useful would this part of the course be to individual students?
3. How would additional needs, if they arose, be supported?
4. What resources were available?

The starting point The starting point needed clarifying as it was agreed that existing skills and knowledge, both individual and shared (or common), were not known, and that assumptions about students' knowledge had been based on previous reported experiences. A great deal of information was already known about each of the course participants, five men and five women, who had all attended sex education within their school setting. Some additional starting information was available, especially the social behaviour of two of the male students. A sexual knowledge assessment would be undertaken initially with each student to give a baseline of knowledge for the group and work out individual learning needs.

Content   The topic areas within the Sexual Knowledge Assessment (Brooke Advisory Centre, 1987) were used as the foundations for an overall plan of subjects to be covered. The number of sessions required to facilitate a topic depended on how long it took the students to work through the subject. The sessions were integrated into the overall college course, continuing for its duration.

Teaching aids   A variety of teaching aids were used and these are described in the References and Useful resources at the end of this chapter. The teaching aids used provided mainly visual images and included slides, pictures and teaching packs designed specifically for people with learning disabilities. Mainstream health promotion resources required adaptation as they are often difficult to interpret.

Teaching resources were reviewed both prior to use and following sessions.

Other people and agencies were used as a valuable input of working experience and to provide a chance to see places such as labour wards (see below).

Evaluation   The course would be evaluated through interview and discussion with each student and through group discussion. This would include evaluating each session and utilising subsequent feedback. The Sexual Knowledge Assessment would be repeated at the end of the course to ascertain individual levels of achievement and identify unmet needs.

Course conclusion   At the end of the course, the students would be given a certificate and a report to be included with their academic report. This would give an account of what work the group had carried out, any individual support or work undertaken and an account of achievement or development. Reports would be individualised with the idea that they could be used for accessing future support, for highlighting other needs and when developing future plans.

Follow up   Needs that could not be met during the session (e.g. disclosure of abuse) would be referred on to an appropriate service with the student's knowledge and consent.

Getting started   It was agreed that the students should be asked about what they would like to include in personal development sessions, based on their previous experiences. Introductory sessions were organised with the students to introduce the themes and the intention to carry out the assessments. The students were asked to work out the ground rules for the group: timing, venue (within the college), confidentiality and group rules (e.g. listening when others were speaking). The group decided that they wanted the following issues incorporated:

- to have a male and a female facilitator
- to talk about themselves
- to listen to what other people said
- to ask questions, if they did not understand something
- to keep what was said during the sessions private, i.e. not for discussion outside
- to have a break for coffee/drinks etc.
- to have the option of individual feedback if someone had a different need (or needs) from the rest of the group
- to meet weekly during term time
- to have some divided sessions: the women did not want to discuss private issues in front of male students (private issues meant that they did not want to talk about their own bodies or personal problems/issues in front of men)
- to carry out the Sexual Knowledge Assessments and for the facilitators to look at the information that was common to the group and feed this information back to the group as a whole.

The facilitators added one other ground rule in terms of confidentiality. This additional ground rule was added in relation to any disclosure that could not be kept completely confidential in relation to risk. For example, if a person needed to talk about something that meant they or someone else was at risk, the facilitators would not be able to keep this completely confidential. Examples of this were illustrated by using pictures and the narrative from *Sex and the 3Rs* (McCarthy and Thompson, 1992).

To help the students to remember the agreements and ground rules, these were developed, with the students, into both word and picture formats. These were revisited from time to time and displayed during each session.

It was important to allow the students to say what they felt had been covered during school (or other) sex education experiences. The range of experience varied between students but a common theme was that they had all worked on understanding their bodies and how they worked. The students agreed that they wished to refresh some of their knowledge but that this did not require to be covered in great detail again. Two people wanted to talk about 'dating' and 'marriage'. Another common theme within the group was 'pregnancy and having babies'. Two of the women wanted to talk about coping with men's behaviour towards them: being touched on occasions, that they had used to consider 'fun' but now found 'annoying'.

Consultation with carers

The college used a newsletter to let parents and carers know what was happening during all aspects of the course. The sex education group was included within routine information. Two responses from carers related to women in the group, raising anxieties for carers of increased vulnerability or the manifestation of inappropriate sexual behaviour.

As the students were over 18 years of age, no one else needed to consent to them attending the group. It was important to acknowledge the anxieties of carers and, after consultation with the students, a letter was sent to all carers giving them an outline of the intended course and inviting them to make further enquiries. The two students whose carers had shown anxiety requested to meet, with their carers, someone from the course to discuss these anxieties.

It is common for parents and carers to have anxieties when considering their child (a person with learning disabilities) as a sexual person. The parents in question were concerned that education would lead to a greater risk of abuse, exploitation and inappropriate sexual behaviour. These are common anxieties expressed by parents (Cooper and Guillebaud, 1999; Drury et al., 2000; Fegan et al., 1993). It is necessary to acknowledge these anxieties and to provide both information (education) and reassurance that the facilitators who are providing support have appropriate knowledge, skills and are 'safe' to work with vulnerable people. It is also important to accept other people's values and beliefs, challenging misconceptions by utilising an appropriate knowledge base: the worker needs to talk from experience utilising information and research available.

A carer is unlikely to feel comfortable with, or trust, a worker who is not honest and open about their experiences. The worker's own values and attitudes, although important, should not be imposed upon others. Account must be taken of a carer's values and beliefs and a balance made with the values, needs and wants of the person with learning disabilities. Parents tend to be concerned with the needs of their own child and may not be able to focus on the needs of a group, or on the views of other parents (Rose and Jones, 1994). Rose and Jones suggest the use of workshops for parents and carers to help in developing understanding and knowledge and they also advocate individual work with parents. A fundamental aspect of providing this support is to recognise the agenda of parents and not only how but why it differs from that of the professional.

In this instance, through several consultations with both sets of carers, it was possible to increase their understanding of the principle that increasing a person's sexual knowledge can lessen the likelihood of the individual becoming a victim of abuse. The individual's sexual behaviour, such as masturbation, is most likely already occurring without the carer's knowledge. Appropriately facilitated sessions should not increase inappropriate sexual behaviour or encourage it to occur.

Perhaps more importantly, the carers were able express their beliefs, attitudes and fears. The opportunity for discussion in the past had not been available, doctors or other professionals providing limited time and information. Other needs of the growing child became more important, especially if ill-health had been a predominant factor.

The teaching aids to be used were also made available for carers to see. Anecdotal accounts of past teaching experiences provided insight into how other people with learning disabilities had made use of information and how problems had been realised, dealt with or referred on for more specific support. These consultations provided the opportunity to assist the carers in being a part of the education process, increased their knowledge and allayed many anxieties about perceived problems.

Assessments The Sexual Knowledge Assessment questionnaire was adapted to incorporate, where necessary, specific questions that were unambiguous, to ensure a consistent way of framing the assessment. The assessment (Brooks Advisory Centre, 1987) utilises pictorial information on which questions are based. Many of the pictures are explicit, and preparation beforehand allowed people to know what they were going to see and what the pictures were intended for. It also provided an opportunity to introduce reassurances that it is alright to feel embarrassed and that this is common when looking at images involving nudity or expression of sexuality. This led on to discussions of pornography (see below).

The course content As stated above, the content of the course was based upon the topic areas within the Sexual Knowledge Assessment. Additional needs were added into these areas as they were realised. The initial assessments indicated the following areas for learning/developmental needs:

- poor knowledge expressed by men about female masturbation
- understanding and concepts about gay or lesbian relationships
- understanding about sexually transmitted diseases and safer sex
- contraception methods, other than women using the pill or men using condoms
- how to gain sexual pleasure, i.e. what parts of the body on a man and a woman can be stimulated to provide sexual pleasure
- other ways of 'having sex', other than heterosexual intercourse
- pregnancy, giving birth and having a baby, based on pictures and line drawings
- non-contact abuse, such as name calling, was poorly identified or defined.

The strengths common to the group in terms of knowledge were as follows:

- all could define contact abuse, be that inappropriate touching or unwanted intercourse
- a common understanding of menstruation, with some variation and accuracy of details
- all wanted to have a relationship (all defined as heterosexual at the time of assessment).

The course ran on a weekly basis and included a half hour break. The group began with a quick ice-breaking session, usually about general personal information or discussion about a news/media story. The session moved on to discussing the topic area, with an outline of what would happen, for example if role play was going to be included, a video was going to be watched and discussed, or a presentation given by another student.

The group was separated into gender groups for particular sessions, where the same topic would be covered. As the facilitator was also of the same gender, there was the opportunity to identify with the facilitator and hopefully feel more confident to share feelings and experiences. The role played by a facilitator is important in terms of providing a credible role model, who must be able to give a clear unbiased perspective. This method of single-sex education groups is discussed in detail by McCarthy (1999). Combined gender groups allowed for discussion to elicit opinions and facilitate debate to develop awareness of how a woman or man might feel or think about certain topics or issues.

Pornography The concept of pornography was raised in relation to the pictorial teaching aids. Following this up allowed people to discuss their feelings and to realise that they did not all share the same views. The facilitators clarified that the tools/aids being used were explicit and that people may feel aroused. However, the difference between these pictures (and other tools) and pornography was that the latter is designed to arouse the onlooker. The pictures and other teaching aids were designed to illustrate information and help people to understand. It was agreed that pornography would not be used in any way during the education process as it could mislead people in terms of accurate information, often relates to fantasy and does not necessarily depict people's choices or preferences in relation to sex.

Teaching aids Teaching resources were reviewed following sessions. If students found something had been difficult to follow or understand, it was repeated, adapting the session in line with the students' comments.

Resources Perhaps the most useful resources were other people and agencies.

A member of a local branch of the National Childbirth Trust (NCT) who was pregnant agreed to join one of the sessions to discuss how she felt about being pregnant, how she felt physically and her expectations about giving birth. She visited again after her baby was born to talk about some of her experiences and brought her baby to the session. This was an invaluable experience for the students, who gained an insight from someone who was able to talk openly not only about the positive aspects of being pregnant and giving birth but also about the unpleasant sensations, feelings of nausea, commencing labour and pain during labour.

Through negotiation with local health visitors, one joined the group to discuss her role in helping to support a new mother. She was also able to arrange for the students to visit the local hospital antenatal and labour suites. Five of the students had the opportunity to be shown around a labour room, where they saw the equipment available, such as pain relief equipment, how the baby is monitored during labour and were able to discuss the role of a birth partner.

Students also visited a local family planning clinic, arranged with the help of a domiciliary family planning nurse. This helped with reinforcing college-based learning about contraception and sexual health. The students were able to meet a doctor and other nurses in a family planning clinic. These professionals were able to give a brief outline of their role and function in this clinic, which again helped to support discussion and recall information during other sessions.

The local Gay Men's Health Advisor supported facilitators with ways of looking at discrimination against gay men and the ways in which gay men obtained support to access health-care advice. This was combined with looking at safer sex within heterosexual, gay and lesbian relationships. It seemed to be more important that the students developed an awareness that sex could be enjoyed safely than that they remembered all the common types of sexually transmitted diseases.

Concluding themes developed by the group The main themes to come out of the group work were as follows:

- You should only do what you want to do, no one should make you.
- Apart from sexual intercourse, there were several ways that two people could enjoy sexual pleasure, through touching, kissing and stimulating each other sexually.
- The use of condoms and dental dams provided protection against sexually transmitted diseases.
- People have 'sexy thoughts' from time to time. These need to be kept private and any sexual expression should be done in private.

- Masturbation should be done privately and you should enjoy it if you want to do it.
- Not everyone was heterosexual (straight).

Social and relationship skills

It was important to frame these sessions within the overall context of the course. Regular liaison and feedback from other course tutors was essential in order to gain a perspective of what experiences the students were having elsewhere.

The students were able to identify different types of social relationship and the context of appropriate behaviours related to these different relationships. Practical experience was gained during most aspects of the course, which in turn helped with discussions. Some of the students were able to identify when they had not behaved in the most appropriate way. Discussion led to the ability to be able to challenge students on how their behaviour conflicted with the role they should have taken in any situation and the role of the other person(s).

An example of this was when one of the men in the group would tickle and touch one of the women during some lunch times. She did not like this attention but had difficulty telling him that she did not wish this to happen. In addition to this, her behaviour almost colluded with his, giving mixed messages. This story was useful in helping to gain insights into other people's views and allowed the woman to express her feelings more clearly. The man had difficulty coming to terms with understanding that his behaviour was not liked by other people. McCarthy (1999) discussed the concepts of men's insights and understanding of how 'the other person' feels; that is, the difficulties learning disabled men seemed to have in appreciating that how they experienced sexual intercourse was not the same as their partner. An analogy of this is how some men with learning disabilities may not appreciate that some of their behaviours may not be perceived the same way by others. They then continue to carry out these behaviours not comprehending the other person's experience.

The behaviour exhibited by this man bordered on offending behaviour and the man was referred on for further support from other learning disability professionals not involved in the group. An individual's concepts, thoughts and behaviours may require to be challenged, perhaps utilising a cognitive behavioural approach conducted by experienced therapists.

Outcomes

Final reports were achieved with input from the students so that they had ownership of the information the reports contained. This was private and personal to the individual concerned. One woman was referred on for sexual health advice. Another woman was referred on for support in relation to bereavement and another woman referred for support following disclosure of potential abuse. One of the men was referred for support with sexualised behaviours, as discussed above, and one other man was referred on for advice and support in relation to sexual health and coming to terms with his sexual orientation.

The students had developed a greater awareness and understanding related to their learning needs identified following the assessment period. They also had the opportunity to develop insight into other services that they could access.

CONCLUSIONS The concept of sexuality needs to be integrated into understanding the needs of a person as a whole and not merely related to a sexual act. Supporters and carers need to take this into account when trying to help. These needs, whether directly related to sexuality or not, require to be thought out by getting to know the individual through appropriate holistic assessment. In the first example discussed in this chapter, John's needs only became apparent as staff got to know him and had improved the daily physical aspects of his care. Although there were concerns about instituting time where John could physically reach to his genitalia, this was a response to a need he had demonstrated and the response could be monitored and adjusted as required. The second example, Jane, was a situation where assumptions were made that only skimmed the surface of her needs. It can be all too easy to make assumptions of what someone needs or wants in an attempt to help them to express their sexuality. Referral to appropriate professionals either for support or for actual specialist intervention is an important aspect of helping. This is also an integral aspect of managing risks relating to sexuality issues such as abuse, exploitation and sexual health. The use of a sex education group is a means of improving the awareness of all aspects of sexuality in a person with a learning difficulty and can identify areas where more specific help is needed.

REFERENCES Aylott J 1999 Is the sexuality of people with learning disabilities being denied? British Journal of Nursing 8(7): 438–442

Brooks Advisory Centre 1987 Sexual knowledge assessment. Brook Publishing, London

Brown H, Turk V 1992 Defining sexual abuse as it affects adults with learning disabilities. Mental Handicap 20: 44–55

Cambridge P, McCarthy M 1997 Developing and implementing sexuality policy for a learning disability provider service. Health and Social Care in the Community 5(4): 227–236

Cooper E, Guillebaud J 1999 Sexuality and disability: a guide for everyday practice. Radcliffe, London

Craft A (ed) 1987 Mental handicap and sexuality: issues and perspectives. Costello Press, London

Dixon H 2002 Picture yourself: a flexible teaching resource for use with people with learning difficulties. Me and Us Publications, Sedbergh, UK

Drury J, Hutchinson L, Wright J 2000 Holding on letting go. Sex, sexuality and people with learning disabilities. Souvenir Press, London

Fegan L, Rauch A, McCarthy W 1993 Sexuality and people with intellectual disability, 2nd edn. McLennan and Petty, Australia

Kempton W 1988 Life horizons I and II. James Stanfield, Santa Barbara, CA

Law Commission 2000 Setting the boundaries: reforming the law on sex offences. Home Office, London

Letts P 1994 Is the law inhibiting relationships?(Law on marriage and sexual relationships in people with learning disabilities.) Community Living 8(1) July 1994 10–11

McCarthy M 1999 Sexuality and women with learning disabilities. Kingsley, London

McCarthy M, Thompson D 1992 Sex and the 3Rs: rights responsibilities and risks. Pavilion, Brighton

O'Sullivan A, Gillies P 1993 You, me and HIV—making sense of safer sex for people with learning difficulties. Daniels, Cambridge

Rose J, Jones C 1994 Working with parents. In: Craft A (ed) Practice issues in sexuality and learning disabilities. Routledge, London

Royal College of Nursing 2000 Sexuality and sexual health in nursing practice. Royal College of Nursing, London

Rutter M 2000 The development of a person. In: Wells D (ed) Caring for sexuality in health and illness. Churchill Livingstone, London

Schwier K, Hingsburger D 2000 Sexuality: your sons and daughters with intellectual disabilities. Kingsley, London

Seedhouse D 1988 Ethics: the heart of health care. Wiley, Chichester

OTHER USEFUL RESOURCES

Becoming a woman. Teaching pack developed by Cooper E. Pavilion, Brighton (*This is a useful resource for teaching both young and older women with learning disabilities about all aspects of menstruation.*)

Condom Teaching Model, produced and distributed by Health Edco, Waco, TX (*This is a latex model penis that can be made erect and to ejaculate. It is relatively life like and a useful aid for teaching people with learning disabilities how to apply and remove condoms safely.*)

Making the change. Teaching pack developed by Cooper E and Welsh R. Pavilion, Brighton (*Another teaching pack developed to help those supporting women with learning disabilities learning about the menopause.*)

4

Mental health and learning disabilities

Colin Beacock

OVERVIEW   Recent reviews of the service needs of people with learning disabilities in the UK have identified a range of deficiencies in health and social care services. One of the areas of greatest concern is in provision of help for those with additional needs related to mental health or social problems. Mental health problems occur in up to 50% of people with learning disabilities, hence the concern. This chapter will examine the specialist mental health needs of people with learning disabilities within the context of evolving services and a growing expertise in meeting the needs of marginalised, vulnerable people in our society. It will also examine a range of policy issues and consider how they will influence this group of people through the services that they receive.

HISTORY OF MENTAL HEALTH AND LEARNING DISABILITY POLICY   Meeting the needs of people with learning disability has proved to be a challenge for society for over 200 years. The roots of the confusion within today's services can be found in the history of mental health and learning disability policy, provision, diagnosis and terminology.

In the late 18th century, the move from a rural to an increasingly urban society, driven by the forces of the Industrial Revolution, created a need to give care and sustenance to the less fortunate members of the population. Where the group of people who we now describe as having 'learning disabilities' were concerned, their destiny was driven as much by the systems and resources of the day as by the nature of their needs. In Britain in the first half of the 19th century, institutional care was the only model available for the most vulnerable and needy groups of people. That meant geographical isolation and block systems of care where individuality was positively discouraged. Individuality was not a commodity that was highly prized in the society of the time. The rights of the individual that now exist have developed during the 20th century. Similarly, individualised assessments of need and the provision of personalised packages of care are concepts of the late 20th century, and even then only in the more affluent societies (Box 4.1).

Box 4.1	**The tale of Christina, a mother in Romania**

The Berlin Wall has fallen; the Chinese are rising against communism and, in our own country, the fall of the despised dictator Ceauscescu has given us all hope of a great future. But here I sit and watch over my son Viorel. He is 20 years old and our home is five floors up in a block of ageing, damp and rowdy flats. But who am I to complain? Viorel makes more noise than anyone does, or at least he used to. We had no doctors to tell us what was wrong with our son. He was just another one of the *handicapatti irrecupabli*. They wanted to take him away from me— he should go to the home, they said. An orphanage; but Viorel is no orphan, he is my son! Five of us share the flat, but Viorel is the one who must be cared for by each of us. If he goes into the home, we will have to pay for his care but never be allowed to see him again. The strain of living with him is too much at times but to live without him, even when he rocks and kicks and screams—may the Lord forgive me for thinking these things.

In the early part of the 19th century, the provisions of the Poor Laws, whereby vagrants and beggars became charges upon the Parish, persisted. Although there is evidence of the establishing of specialist private homes for 'idiots' and 'imbeciles', the terminology of the period for people with learning disability, most in this group got whatever service they could from Poor Law institutions, primarily the workhouse. The alternative was a public lunatic asylum. These were being established by 1880, at an increasing rate across the whole of the country and were geared to providing for the needs of those who were mentally ill. Although it was recognised that people with learning disabilities were different from the mentally ill, or 'lunatics', there was only one system for the care of both groups. It was realised that the 'idiots and imbeciles' had no prospect of being 'cured'. The Idiots Act (1886) and the Lunacy Act (1891) made it possible legally to certify people separately as idiots or imbeciles and this enabled specialist asylums to be created for their care. This required a proper assessment to identify this group. Because they could not be 'rehabilitated', and were unlikely to make any significant contribution to the national product of an industrialised society, people with learning disabilities, or mental deficiency, began to be perceived as a problem. Thomson (1998, p 13) summarised this situation:

> Although the emergence of the charitable idiot asylums was undoubtedly important in creating a model of specialised residential care, their history cannot fully explain why mental deficiency became to be seen as such a significant problem by the end of the century. Their problems were not insurmountable, they could be solved by being more selective over the types of cases they accepted, and by leaving the chronic to be provided for elsewhere. Whereas the seemingly bottomless pit of public lunatic asylums provision created a vicious circle of escalating demand for further institutional care, a comparable role

cannot be attributed to idiot asylums, whose growth was always restrained by their charitable status and funding. Instead, to understand why mental deficiency became a major social problem one needs to look at the way it became defined as a management problem which overlapped a range of institutional settings, including schools, workhouses, lunatic asylums, prisons, and inebriate reformatories.

In a society that valued order and predictability, it was a serious disadvantage to be defined as difficult to provide for and not productive. Furthermore, as the Idiots Act and Lunacy Act reflect, there was an increasing recognition in late Victorian society that it was inappropriate to provide care for this group of people in the company of the mentally ill, nor was it appropriate that they should be covered by the provisions of legislation for the poor. Whereas mental illness was perceived to be a fairly simple concept, and its victims could be cared for in the provisions of the County or Metropolitan Asylum system, here was a group of people who did not fit comfortably into any single social system, as Thomson (1998) described.

As late Victorian society sought to improve the quality of life for citizens by increasing regulation and control, it became increasingly important to fit comfortably into a specific group as politicians began to legislate for the underprivileged. People who did not fit, or who had a complexity of needs, were difficult to legislate and provide for. The general lack of distinction between those with mental health needs and those with learning disabilities, and the services they received, is partly the reason why confusion amongst politicians, practitioners and the general public has proliferated. If people with mental health needs are marginalised within society, then those people who are additionally, and primarily, suffering from some form of learning disability are doubly disadvantaged. As it was in the late Victorian era, so it is today.

Policy at the start of the 21st century

A review of the quality of services for people with learning disabilities across England was conducted by the Department of Health in 1999. The resulting report, *Facing the facts* (Department of Health, 1999a), identified a range of deficiencies in health and social care services. One of the areas of greatest concern was in services for people with additional needs related to mental health or social problems. In summarising the outcomes of their research, the project team stated that (Department of Health, 1999a, p 20):

> In both the field work visits and questionnaires, concerns were expressed about services—most especially health services—for people with additional needs related to mental health or a variety of social problems. These are people who may often challenge society or services—whether because of mental illness, personality disorder,

offending behaviour, drug or alcohol abuse, or other social problems—
and who might fall through the net for one reason or another. For
instance, in one area, there was said to be no specialist service available
for people with dual diagnosis of learning disability and mental health
problems, while in another, generic services (of various kinds) were
said to be inadequately resourced, and staff inadequately trained.

The research was wide and thorough, so there is no reason to believe that
this situation only pertains in particular localities. Indeed the prevalence
of mental health problems in people who have learning disabilities is
described in another document of that same year, *Once a day* (Department
of Health, 1999b, p 17):

> Mental health problems, including challenging behaviour, occur in
> up to 50% of people with learning disabilities. Depression and with-
> drawal are frequently not diagnosed or treated. The prescription of
> psychotropic medication should be based on the advice of a psych-
> iatrist with special knowledge of learning disabilities.

Given that mental health needs are so frequently associated with a
learning disability, it might be surprising to learn that the guidance in
Once a day is aimed at the primary health-care team and most especially
at GPs. Clearly, if there is so much ignorance of the specialist health-care
needs of people with learning disabilities that GPs, the cornerstone of
our primary care services, need to have specific guidance on the subject,
there has to be some reasoning behind that situation.

DEFINING MENTAL ILLNESS AND LEARNING DISABILITIES

What the Victorians began, society has continued to this day. Diagnosis,
classification and definitions are crucial because they determine a
person's eligibility to a service and they may well have implications
for that person's capacity to make meaningful choices about their lives.
They may also determine a person's culpability at law when they have
committed a crime or unlawful act. The definitions we use to determine and describe a learning disability and a mental health illness are
crucial to our acknowledgement of special needs. If having a mental
health problem *and* a learning disability creates additional complications
for people who are already at the margins of society, then the definitions of mental illnesses and associated conditions can only serve to
complicate matters further.

Mental illness

As a basic guide, contemporary thinking has it that there are two main
forms of mental illness: neurosis and psychosis. The diagnostic difficulties and lack of specificity in defining these conditions is well summarised by the definitions offered in *Tabers cyclopedic medical dictionary*
(Thomas et al., 1993).

Neurosis. Thomas et al. (1993) define this (p 1303) as follows:

> The definition of this term is controversial. Some feel that its use should be limited to describing an unpleasant mental symptom in an individual with intact reality testing: others would have it apply to the etiological process, i.e., unconscious conflict that arouses anxiety and leads to maladaptive use of defensive mechanisms that result in symptom formation. Alternatively, some consider the neuroses to have a physical basis. To further confuse this picture, some would entirely abandon the terms neurosis and psychoneurosis and replace them with anxiety disorders (panic states, phobias, and obsessive-compulsive neuroses) and somataform disorders (hysteria, conversion symptoms, and hypochondriasis).

Psychosis. Thomas et al. (1993, p 1631) define this as:

> A term formerly applied to any mental disorder, but now generally restricted to those disturbances of such magnitude that there is personality disintegration and loss of contact with reality. The disturbances are of psychogenic origin … or clearly defined physical causes or structural change to the brain. They are usually characterised by delusions and hallucinations and hospitalisation is generally required.

This condition is manifest in the behaviour, emotional reaction and ideation of the patient, who fails to mirror reality as it is, reacts erroneously to it, and builds up false concepts regarding it. Behaviour responses are peculiar, abnormal, inefficient or definitely antisocial.

Mental illness in those with learning disability

When considering the needs of a person with learning disability who may also have some form of mental health need, it can be crucial to determine which set of needs is of primary importance. The critical consideration of whether or not a learning disability is a form of psychiatric disorder is exemplified by recent attempts to legislate for the needs of people with mental health needs. The first attempt to legislate specifically for the needs of people with learning disabilities and mental illness was, arguably, the Mental Health Act 1959 (Department of Health and Welsh Office, 1959). By the late 1970s, however, that Act was felt to be overly prescriptive, too medically dominated and in need of revision. The most recent legislation on mental health came onto the statute books in the form of the Mental Health Act 1983 (Department of Health and Welsh Office, 1983). At the time of writing in late 2001, that legislation is still current in England and Wales. In this Act, the term 'mental disorder' is crucial in determining whether or not a person would be subject to the Act and is used to describe mental illness, arrested or incomplete development of mind, psychopathic disorder and any other disorder or disability of mind.

The all-embracing nature of this description raises problems in determining whether or not a person with learning disabilities should be subject to the orders of the Mental Health Act. There is some difficulty in determining the nature of 'arrested' or 'incomplete' development of mind as a learning disability and the Act goes on to describe four specific categories for the classification of mental disorders, two of which have relevance specifically for people with learning disabilities. These are (Department of Health and Welsh Office, 1983, s1 (2)):

Mental impairment.   '... a state of arrested or incomplete development of mind not amounting to severe mental impairment which includes significant impairment of intelligence and social functioning and is associated with abnormally aggressive or seriously irresponsible conduct on the part of the person.'

Severe mental impairment.   '... A state of arrested or incomplete development of mind which includes severe mental impairment of intelligence and social functioning and is associated with abnormally aggressive or seriously irresponsible conduct on the part of the person concerned.'

Assessment of the degree of impairment   The differential between the definition of 'mental' and 'severe mental' impairment is one of degree. Unlike the differentiation between neurosis and psychosis, this distinction is merely determined by the intensity of a range of symptoms or behaviours within a central definition. What we have is a situation wherein the level of impairment is more crucial than the nature of the problems that give rise to it, and this is acknowledged by the Mental Health Act 1983 when it states (s10): 'This distinction between the two degrees of mental impairment is important because there are differences in the grounds on which patients can be detained, or have their detention renewed, if they suffer from severe mental impairment as opposed to mental impairment' (Department of Health and Welsh Office, 1983).

Consequently, abnormally aggressive or seriously irresponsible conduct can lead to persons with a learning disability being subject to an Act under which they might lose their liberty and freedom. The term 'challenging behaviour' is widely used to describe a range of actions on the part of a person with a learning disability that challenge the understanding and resources of other people. This description is generally one that is imposed upon the person by those who have no experience of having a learning disability; the cause of the challenging behaviour might be anything ranging from a mental health problem to lack of social skills development or to cognitive impairment. Nonetheless, because of the nature of the behaviours they display, if that person has a prior diagnosis of mental impairment, they may be considered to be abnormally aggressive, seriously irresponsible or even mentally ill, thus making them subject to the provisions of the Mental Health Act. The end result is that a learning disability, whatever its cause, is sufficient for a person to be subject to the provisions of the Mental Health Act.

Role of psychiatrists

Any confusion that might have existed about the differential between mental health needs and learning disabilities is further compounded by the role played by psychiatrists in determining whether or not a person with learning disabilities should be subject to the Act. The Mental Health Act *Code of practice* (Department of Health and Welsh Office, 1999) suggests (s30.4) that 'No patient should be classified under the Act as mentally impaired or severely mentally impaired without an assessment by a consultant psychiatrist in learn-ing disabilities and a formal psychological assessment. This assessment should be part of a complete appraisal by medical, nursing, social work and psychology professionals with experience in learning disabilities ...'

Even though this guidance offers an opportunity for other professional opinions to be involved in the process of assessment, it is apparent that the only compulsory element required is the opinion of the psychiatrist. When first published, the Mental Health Act 1983 attracted considerable criticism for the manner in which it appeared to cement the central importance of medical opinion above all others.

Review of the Mental Health Act

In much the same way that the Mental Health Act of 1959 was previously deemed to be requiring of review, so the 1983 Act was subject to review and a report was subsequently published in 1999 (Department of Health, 1999c). The specific needs of people with learning disabilities were considered within this process and it was stated within the report (p 41, s4.19) that:

> We have received clear submissions, on behalf of both those with learning disabilities and those who care for them, to the effect that a Mental Health Act is not the appropriate vehicle for the provision of such a framework. The principle reasons include:
>
> i) the care and support required in the case of learning disability extends much further than treatment for mental disorder;
> ii) people with a learning disability do not, on the whole, require medical treatment for mental disorder;
> iii) inclusion within a mental health act is thought to be stigmatising for the patient and for the family;
> iv) the need for care and support in the case of learning disability is typically long standing, while for mental illness needs may fluctuate;
> v) the formal structure required for the imposition of compulsion in the case of mental disorder would not be appropriate to learning disability.

On the basis of these points, it seems clear that to subject someone to the provisions of the Mental Health Act on the basis that they have a learning disability is acknowledged as being inappropriate. It would also appear that there is a real need to consider someone with learning disabilities as being of the same status as any other citizen in our society, and that the authority of mental health legislation should only be applied if that person is identified as having some form of mental illness, rather than impairment, as described by the Mental Health Act 1983.

Consent and rights   What emerges is that the provisions of the Mental Health Act have been used for people with a learning disability as a means of protecting their rights, related to the capacity to give informed consent, rather than their mental health state. If you or I were to be assessed within the provisions of the Act, we would not first be assessed as to whether or not we had a learning disability. It is evident that, in effect, the powers of the Mental Health Act have been applied to enable professionals to reinforce their ability to determine what would constitute the best interests of a person with learning disabilities where that person does not have the capacity to give informed consent. This was highlighted by a legal case, which has become known as *Bournewood* (1998), whereby a health authority sought a legal ruling as to whether or not a psychiatrist could make patients with learning disabilities subject to the Mental Health Act as a means of ensuring their protection on the basis of their inability to give informed consent and to ensure that the practitioner could determine their best interests. Many of these issues have been addressed in a government discussion document called *Who decides* (Lord Chancellor's Department, 1997) but as yet this has not given rise to the enactment of any new legislation that will enable better representation of those people who cannot give informed consent. Recognising these factors, in addition to those raised through submissions by and on behalf of people with a learning disability, the Expert Committee (Department of Health, 1999c) nonetheless decided (p 42, s4.20):

> While we appreciate the strength of this reasoning and fully support the argument that a new comprehensive statutory framework is required, we nonetheless do not wish to see learning disabilities excluded from any new Mental Health Act. In the first place we consider it important to ensure that assessment, under compulsion if necessary, is available for those with a learning disability and co-occurring mental illness. Secondly, there may be those with a learning disability who display challenging behaviour, including self-harm, for whom care and treatment under the framework provided by the Mental Health Act is appropriate.

Furthermore, in respect of *Bournewood* and similar circumstances, the Expert Committee (Department of Health, 1999c, p 42, s4.22) felt:

> Unfortunately we now realise that no legislative proposals from Who Decides? will emerge in the near future. We are therefore left with the possibility that there may be people with learning disability and long-term incapacity who the law may regard as detained, albeit under common law not the Mental Health Act, and for whom no proper safeguards exist. In these circumstances such people may have to enter into long-term compulsory care and treatment under the new mental health legislation in order to acquire the required safeguards, even if they have a learning disability alone and no mental illness. ... For the reasons stated above we do not think people who require care and treatment for their learning disabilities should be provided for under a Mental Health Act designed primarily for those with other forms of mental disorder.

What emerges, therefore, is a system in which there is a perverse incentive for people with a learning disability to be made subject to an inappropriate form of legislation as a means of protecting their rights. The conclusion must be drawn that the confusion and lack of understanding amongst GPs, as indicated within *Once a day* (Department of Health, 1999b), and the inconsistencies in service quality, described within *Facing the facts* (Department of Health, 1999a), are entirely consistent with other parts of our system of care. Not only is there a general lack of understanding of the personal and clinical needs of people with learning disabilities, but where this is complicated by a diagnosis of mental illness, they are caught up in a situation where confusion about their primary diagnosis can result in them being subject to an utterly inappropriate form of legislation.

MAKING SENSE OF THE CONFUSION: DEVELOPING PROFESSIONAL PRACTICE

The definitions offered previously of neurosis and psychosis referred to the 'controversial' nature of descriptions of conditions and to the fact that terminologies have changed to such a degree that the entire classification of some disorders has been altered. The authors of these definitions indicated the lack of explicit agreement that exists in the field of psychiatry about the disorders described. Given the confusion and political atmosphere that surrounds the very nature of diagnoses of both mental illness and learning disabilities, creating operational procedures and some form of guidance for practitioners poses problems. The salient feature appears to be the ability to differentiate behaviours and symptoms, when both have a wide spectrum and these overlap in places. Some of the dilemmas involved in trying to describe how these main forms of mental illness vary are covered by May and Baker (1977, p 8) in their guide for GPs:

> In broad differential classification of mental illness, setting aside the organic states which are classified on the basis of the morbid process, it is generally said that the neurotic has insight into or understanding of his illness, whereas the psychotic has not. Unfortunately for this convenient distinction, there are neurotics such as hysterics who have little insight and psychotics, such as some patients with endogenous depression or early schizophrenia, who do realise that they are ill. However, it is usual for a psychosis to distort the whole personality and the patient becomes unable to distinguish between his delusions and hallucinations and reality, whereas the neurotic can distinguish between his morbid experiences and reality ... Perhaps the most useful division between the neuroses and the psychoses is the viewing of neurotic symptomatology as an exaggeration and prolongation of normal behaviour under stress, whereas psychotic behaviour is bizarre and shows such distortion of reality as to put it outside the normal range of experience.

Given the previous references in this chapter to the crucial role that GPs will play in developing community-based services for people with learning disabilities and their need for mainstream NHS primary care services, this guidance is useful because it illustrates the level of understanding that many GPs have of mental illnesses. In suggesting that classification of mental illnesses was a useful enterprise because it enabled more accurate diagnosis and treatment, the guide went on to demonstrate a useful classification for family doctors (May and Baker, 1977, p 9):

1) Subnormal intellectual endowment (mental defect).
2) The neuroses:
    a) anxiety states including phobias
    b) hysterical conversion states
    c) obsessional/compulsive neurosis
    d) reactive or neurotic depression
    e) anorexia nervosa.
3) Sexual Problems and Deviations, many of which have their basis in neurotic difficulties.
4) Alcoholism and Drug Addiction.
5) Psychopathic States in which antisocial behaviour and conduct is the predominant manifestation.
6) Psychosomatic Disorders where it is considered that psychological factors play an important role in the production of a physical lesion, e.g. peptic ulcer, skin conditions such as eczema and psoriasis.
7) The psychoses:
    a) functional psychoses in which so far there has been no evidence of a specific lesion in the nervous system to account for the grossly disturbed functioning,
        i) Manic—Depressive or affective Psychosis
        ii) Schizophrenia
        iii) Schizo—affective psychosis in which both symptoms of schizophrenia and affective psychosis are present.

b) organic psychosis in which the psychiatric illness is a result of cerebral or generalised systemic physical disease. This covers a wide group of conditions ranging from syphilis and carcinoma to the delirium of pneumonia.

8) Child Psychiatry.

Children tend to have similar psychiatric conditions to adults, although psychosis is comparatively rare. However, the manifestations and unique problems of the children require a rather different approach. This is an area, which is of special importance to the family doctor.

Notwithstanding the terminology of the day, it is perhaps interesting that the list should commence with 'subnormal intellectual endowment'. That is to say, learning disability, as we now would term it, was perceived to be one of a number of psychiatric disorders. The text was written in the first edition in 1966 and amended in 1977; it was valued by GPs and GP students until the late 1980s. It should come as no surprise that there is still some confusion as to the status of people with learning disabilities and their mental health needs, given the recent nature of this kind of thinking.

DEFINING MENTAL HEALTH NEEDS IN PEOPLE WITH LEARNING DISABILITIES

A guide to the assessment of health needs in people with a learning disability (Matthews, 1996, p 25) states, 'Research would suggest that mental health problems are a major issue for people with learning disabilities. Most frequently the existence of such problems is seen in behavioural patterns. In people with learning disabilities however these patterns may be due to other things, but that question is a matter for those qualified to make a differential diagnosis.' This comment highlights several points. First, the level of diagnosed mental illness is higher in people with learning disabilities than in other groups of people. Second, there are reasons why this should be, which do not apply in other groups in society. Third, the establishing of a form of diagnosis has been historically more crucial to people with learning disabilities than any other group of vulnerable people in our society, and the qualification to make that diagnosis has reinforced the power and influence of professional practitioners over the lives of people in their care.

The effect of institutionalisation

In order to understand why diagnosis is such a complex issue, it is necessary to consider the origins of today's services for people with learning disabilities, especially since the White Paper *Better services for the mentally handicapped* (Department of Health and Social Security, 1972). It was the case, when this White Paper was written, that there were 57 000 beds for people who were living in long-stay hospitals for the mentally handicapped. The White Paper set an objective of reducing those beds to less than 5000, and that figure had been almost achieved by 1997. One of the unfortunate effects of this historical model of care, which we chose to use for people with learning disabilities, was institutional-isation. The system of care in these establishments was based upon mass and congregate living. The establishments were not geared to individual but to collective needs of the patient population. Consequently, the methods of management were structured and routine, rather than flex-ible and adaptable, and the people who lived and worked in these settings developed coping strategies that were driven by the need to conform to that regimen. Lack of stimulation and a failure to provide alternative models of behaviour resulted in patients adopting socially inappropriate behaviours. Congregate living with high levels of expos-ure to paternalistic/maternalistic methods of care tended to increase dependence upon a centralised structure in which the doctor was a dominant force. This dominance led to a medical model of care being offered in remote hospitalised services, which were usually single-sex facilities. The result has been generations of disempowered people who were truly marginalised from the main assets of societal living. It has also meant that the behaviours of this group of people were driven by norms that were separate from those of a normal social group, and very often highly inappropriate. The inappropriateness of these behav-iours further served to reinforce society's negative perceptions of the worth and needs of this group of vulnerable people, creating a self-fulfilling cycle of dependency and poor quality of services. Furthermore, the constant reinforcement of inappropriate and routine behaviours in an institutional system of care, in which education, treatment and ther-apy is of less relevance than containment and conformity, led to a con-dition that may be termed 'institutional neurosis' (Box 4.2). By this, it is meant that the behaviours have become so deep-seated in the mental mechanisms of the person that they have become neurotic in their nature. One major outcome of a system of care that was intended to assist people with learning disabilities, therefore, has been to establish and reinforce a set of behaviours that re-emphasised the need for that person to remain in institutional care, for their own protection and for the protec-tion of other members of society. Another major outcome has been to establish a second set of problem behaviours, which overlie the initial diagnosis of learning disability and serve to disadvantage the person still further. That these behaviours should manifest themselves in such a way that they appear to represent some form of mental illness may have served to reinforce the value of psychiatry in a service for people with learning disabilities. What has clearly happened is that a vulnerable group of people has been subjected to a system of care and a lifestyle that has promoted the development of a secondary diagnosis of mental illness in many. It has also given rise to a system where management of behaviours has focussed on prescription of medications, rather than re-education and social therapies (Box 4.2).

| Box 4.2 | **Arthur** |

I saw my case notes the other day. I sneaked into the office whilst the Charge Nurse was playing snooker. I knew they had been talking about me; the doctor had called me into the office and listened to my chest, just like he did last year. The usual stuff: 'Sit down Arthur, let's have a look in your ears, let's have a look at your chest; aye, you'll do!'

They do not know I can read. There is nothing much to read on here anyway. I have been in here since Mum died and I have not spoken to them since the day they brought me here 8 years ago. I never have and I never will. Nobody asked me if I wanted to come here. Nobody cares. The staff never hurt me but they don't love me like my Mum did.

We had no visitors, me and my Mum, not after Uncle Reg died and he was Mum's only brother. Lovely and quiet out there on the fen; we had to keep things quiet she said, nobody should know I was here. My Dad was a pilot but he never came back from the War; at least not to our house anyway. Best thing my Mum ever did was teach me to read. She had to; said she couldn't send me to school because I was a spastic and spastics do not go to school. You just stay there Arthur and listen to the wireless, Don't try to walk too far, you'll fall over! They have never even asked if I can read or write, and I do not suppose they would understand if I tried to tell them. Only Mum could understand me. I talk funny, you see.

It is a strange thing, me choosing not to talk and keeping out of the way of folks. They call it 'reactive depression'. Something to do with my Mum dying, the psychiatrists say. I am on tablets for it, have been since I came in here. They are not really for my illness but to help me stay calm. They say. I have to be careful or I get sunburnt very easily when I sit in the garden. But I usually keep them under my tongue and spit them out. Nobody notices after medicines because that is when they open the toilets and they cannot keep an eye on all of us, can they? Straight down the pan they goes! And you know what the Charge Nurse says 'Good old Arthur, bowels as regular as clockwork!'

My nursing case notes are funny, though; they just say;

17/10/57 Admitted from home in the care of the Borough Council. (See main notes in Medical Records for family history.) Withdrawn and sullen on examination. Mute child of 12 years (?) with unsteady gait arising from cerebral palsy. Chest fields appear clear. No obvious illness or infestation.

15/10/58 Remains the same
16/10/59 Remains the same
17/10/60 Remains the same
18/10/61 Remains the same
19/10/62 Remains the same
12/10/63 Remains the same
13/10/64 Remains the same
17/10/65 Remains the same

Some things never change! Still, they are talking about bringing in a telly next week for the World Cup Final so the staff can watch it. I ain't never seen a telly but we might get a chance to watch if we keep quiet—I know I will! So long as I am not too depressed!

As Matthews (1996) stated, research has shown that the incidence of mental illness in people with learning disabilities is higher than in the normal population. However, the fact that many of the behaviours demonstrated by this group of people may be the result of institutionalisation, and the behaviours in themselves challenge our resources and capacities, further complicates that research. Turner and Moss (1996, p 440) describe how:

> Studies which include behaviour disorders as psychiatric problems result in high prevalence rates of up to 60% in hospital populations. ... However, if people [are considered] whose only form of disorder is a behavioural disorder, then the prevalence of psychosis and neurosis combined appears to be as low as 8–10%. ... This confusion has been exacerbated by the fact that challenging behaviours are the most common reason for which people with learning disabilities are referred to a psychiatrist, accounting for a third of admissions from the community. ... However, these problems are often long-term behaviour patterns, rather than illnesses showing a predictable time course. As such they often do not fit the established criteria for diagnosable psychiatric conditions. ...

Diagnosing mental illness

Given the confusion that can arise from attempting to differentiate between a behavioural disorder and a psychiatric illness, it seems reasonable to assume that many people with learning disabilities have been unnecessarily given a secondary diagnosis of mental illness. With this in mind, Matthews (1996) sought instead to direct the assessment of health care for a person with learning disabilities towards the outward symptoms which might indicate that they have some form of mental health need. The following symptoms are common behaviours in people with learning disabilities but which Matthews (1996) suggests may be indicative of mental ill health:

- frequent emotional distress
- apparently irrational mood swings
- altered perceptions
- confusional state
- irrational fears and anxieties
- obsessions
- psychosomatic symptoms, which carers often interpret as something that is being 'put on'.

By adopting a symptomatic, rather than diagnostic approach to these areas of health-care need, we are more likely to improve our ability to describe behaviours. Using this approach, assessment of needs tends to orientate providers more towards an individualised care programme, in which the outcomes are in keeping with a variety of complex needs, rather than establishing a diagnosis that leads to a set pattern of interventions, including a medical regimen of care. In this way, the disorder is interpreted as much in terms of a quality of life issue as it is a medical condition or a set of challenging behaviours.

However, where a person has a serious form of mental illness that presents together with a learning disability, it is important that they receive an appropriate regimen of treatment; here a clinical diagnosis is crucial in getting that treatment. The diagnostic process must be suitable for the lifestyle of the individual. The skills and capacities of staff who care for this client group are crucial, therefore, for diagnosis and assessment of behaviours. Quigley et al. (2001) described how staff in a service for people with learning disabilities were able to identify symptoms that were typical of mental health need as, in fact, behaviours, particularly where they had received training in the subject. Moreover, nursing staff were far more able to recognise and describe symptoms of anxiety, depression and psychosis. Given the previously acknowledged problems in making concrete diagnoses of mental illnesses, it seems likely that staff competence will have influenced the number of people with learning disabilities who had secondary or primary diagnoses of identified mental illness. Equally, assessment methodologies may not be sufficiently flexible to reflect the complexity of people with learning disabilities. Quigley et al. (2001), when considering the relationship between assessment methodologies, abilities of care staff to identify symptoms and the mental health needs of people with learning disability, described this (p 242):

> Meins (1995) examined depression in clients with learning disability and found that 55% of symptoms in the mild group and 83% of symptoms in the severe group were not included in DSM-III-R [an assessment tool]. These symptoms included self-injury, aggression, screaming and stereotyped behaviours ... Moss (1996), in examining the validity of the diagnosis of schizophrenia based on the PAS-ADD [an assessment tool], themselves concluded that the symptoms displayed, while clearly psychotic, may not be sufficient under standardised criteria to be classified with a diagnosis of schizophrenia.

It seems reasonable, therefore, to assume that the prevalence of mental health problems in people with learning disabilities is under-reported. If this is taken in conjunction with the fact that carers may well be inclined to interpret and treat behaviours, rather than symptoms, the cause of a good deal of confusion and inconsistency amongst practitioners and service providers is clearly established.

MEETING THE MENTAL HEALTH NEEDS OF PEOPLE WITH LEARNING DISABILITIES

It is unreasonable and unproductive to expect that an individual with learning difficulties can adapt to a system of care that may be inappropriate, given their intellectual impairment and developmental needs. Turner and Moss (1996, p 441) considered this aspect:

> At the present time ... the evidence indicates that the prevalence of mental illness in people with leaning disability is at least as high as in

the general population. For a person with a learning disability, whose adaptive skills may already be limited, an additional mental illness may herald a move to a more congregate level of care. Taken together, the joint contributions of mental illness and learning disability point to a group of individuals whose need for support is likely to be considerable, and whose quality of life will remain seriously impaired if their psychiatric problems are not effectively diagnosed and treated.

The matter of how we choose to interpret and respond to behaviours in people with learning disabilities is considered by Gear et al. (2000). In discussing the range of theories that inform our thinking about the behaviours of others and the subsequent interventions offered to remedy, in others, behaviours which are unacceptable or inappropriate to ourselves, they state (p 28):

> The more conscious we become of the variety of theories available to us, the better position we are in to be conscious of the theories that inform our actions. More importantly, we may then become more aware of their implications for the people we are trying to help.

> We can choose to offer people tools, skills and choices or we can choose to intervene in more or less controlling ways. We can condition or 'shape' or we can enable development and change (or both) in differing degrees. How we have been taught, or choose, to view people and their behaviour will affect how we behave in return, the kinds of interventions (if any) we are likely to make and how successful those interventions are likely to be.

The range and nature of interventions that are practised with people who exhibit disturbed or challenging behaviours should be informed by a theoretical knowledge, and the effects of such interventions should be subject to research. As already established, the way in which these behaviours are described, and how we value the people who display them, influence treatment and what interventions are offered. Gear et al. (2000, p 77) described a range of such interventions and therapies:

- non-violent (compassionate) communication
- arts therapies
- chemotherapy and physical treatments
- gentle teaching
- structured teaching
- behavioural interventions
- cognitive behavioural interventions.

In doing so, it is perhaps indicative of the attitude of these authors that they described the behaviours of their client group as behavioural distress rather than mental illness or challenging behaviours. It appears, therefore, that they are adopting a more person-centred approach and perceiving the problem from the perspective of the person they are seeking to help. This illustrates the relevance of the attitude, theory and relationship from which the carer or therapist is working when describing the condition. It follows from this, however, that the interventions practised will largely be determined by how the person making the diagnosis perceives the problem and relates to their client. It also serves to reinforce an argument for using multidisciplinary assessment of needs when trying to establish a holistic programme of care for a person with learning disabilities, regardless of whether they have a secondary diagnosis or not. It also follows that a range of other factors can influence a decision on how to treat any person with a mental disorder and can give rise to some interventions being used in preference to others, regardless of their suitability or clinical efficacy. This is explained by Turkistani (2000, p 132):

> Overuse of chemotherapy at the present time arises from a number of different factors; for example, psychological treatments are time-consuming and the waiting list to see a therapist may be several months; consequently family doctors and psychiatrists sometimes prescribe medication while patients are waiting for appointments with therapists. Another factor is that some patients prefer pharmacotherapy as they have greater faith in medication than in therapies. Also, in developing countries pharmacotherapy is often the main, if not the only, treatment in the field of psychiatry, as the number of therapists is very few and psychotherapy is time-consuming and potentially expensive for providers of health services (Box 4.3).

Box 4.3	**Christina and Viorel cont.**

Then the men from the West came. We went to their clinic; we took Viorel out of the flat for the first time in 5 years, travelled 150 kilometers in our friend's car. We had to sell our store of Kent cigarettes to get enough ration tokens to buy the petrol and we had to queue for 3 hours and bribe the man at the garage to get our supply. But we did it. And for what?

They told us he has autism. That he needs stimulation and consistency and a good diet and opportunities for choice. That he needs day care and a chance to develop other relationships and to be challenged. But here in Brasov, in the heart of the mountains with no services and no help? With no money, no support and no one to even advise us?

They gave us a bottle of tablets to help to control his behaviour. And he has taken them. And now he sits there and does not seem to know I am here. No more noise, but no more smiles. He is difficult to move now and difficult to feed and I have only been giving him the tablets for 4 days but they have all gone. What will I do now that they are gone? He looks so ill. Did they say one a day or one a week, I could not be sure.

I pray to God that I have heard them correctly and I pray to God that I can keep going. Sometimes I hear voices and they tell me to do terrible things. I do not want to do it but they insist. So strong; so loud; so often. No one should die for the love of their child, I tell myself. My husband says that I imagine these things, that soon we will have the gas and electricity on again and that the water will be on during the day, and that we will be able to care for Viorel better. But he does not say these things when he drinks, and he drinks a lot. Our other sons do not come home anymore. The youngest is only 14 but he stays in the streets; he does not come home. I should not have let them talk me into having the abortion. My sisters believe I am mad, and now I begin to wonder if I am. When will the sun shine again?

It can be seen that there is a commonality between the institutional systems of care in the UK and the care of people in developing countries: limited choice; too few specialist resources; ease of diagnosis when there are limited treatments. There are familiar tones in all these points. Nonetheless, as person-centred, multidisciplinary care is growing, so the range of options in treatment and therapy has begun to influence policy development. There can be no doubt, however, that the emergence of alternative forms of treatment and intervention has made the task of providing for the mental health needs of people with learning disabilities an increasing burden for practitioners and managers. This situation is further exacerbated because it is accompanied by raised expectations and a growing unwillingness to accept that these mental health conditions are incurable.

POLICY DEVELOPMENT FOR PEOPLE WITH LEARNING DISABILITIES AND MENTAL HEALTH NEEDS

Facing the facts (Department of Health, 1999a) was written against a background of increasing awareness of the benefits of community-based services for people with a learning disability. Humanist philosophies in the 1960s and normalist philosophies in the 1970s and 1980s have done much to shape the thinking and attitude of strategic planners. These philosophies, together with a series of inquiries into scandalous systems of care, have also given rise to an appreciation of the inappropriateness of institutional systems of care. Subsequently, new policy guidance in England and Wales, *Valuing people* (Department of Health, 2001), and Scotland, *The same as you?* (Scottish Executive, 2000), have accelerated the closure of the last of the long-stay hospital beds for people with learning disabilities in these countries and emphasised the need for greater choice, independence, rights and inclusion for people with a learning disability. The preferred model of care for the vast majority of the client group is supported living in small group or individual community-based homes.

What has also emerged is an increasing awareness that people with learning disabilities should utilise and benefit from the same mainstream health-care services as everyone else, including specialist mental health services. However, the backbone of future provision for this group of people will be primary care, hence the concerns about the levels of understanding of GPs and other primary care practitioners about the mental health needs of people with a learning disability. These professionals will have a crucial role in determining access to specialist and community-based services. *Valuing people* (Department of Health, 2001) identified six areas of specialist need in which practitioners should focus their efforts in developing practice and establishing more appropriate systems of care. These included mental health needs and accessing health-care services. This indicates that there is now no need for a separate mental health policy for people with learning disabilities. It is the justifiable expectation of this group to benefit from and be included within all relevant policy and legislation as equal and valued members of society. Currently, the key platform for mental health policy in England and Wales is the national service framework for mental health (Department of Health, 1999d). Although this does not have recommendations specific to the needs of people with learning disabilities and mental health needs, the main areas for raising standards should address a great many of their requirements where they are applied to people with learning disabilities:

- mental health promotion
- primary care and access to services
- effective services for people with severe mental illness
- caring about carers
- preventing suicide.

CONCLUSION Is helping people with learning disabilities and mental health needs a part of our service or a service apart? Why should we be surprised that GPs and other healthcare practitioners are unaware of the specialist health-care needs of this group of people? Why should it have been so remarkable that services in one area should be so much poorer than in another? *Facing the facts* (Department of Health, 1999a) served only to affirm what has been known for many years: people with learning disabilities are caught in a self-fulfilling circle of low expectations, inappropriate and negative social perceptions and blatant ignorance as to their personal needs. Where there is positive intent, society too often adopts a maternalistic/paternalistic approach, choosing to smother potential rather than challenging and enabling.

Why should GPs be any different from anyone else? One good reason is because 90% of people with learning disabilities do not live in institutions, nor have they ever done so. How have they been obtaining services? Who has been offering care to the person who is isolated at home with their family or living in a small group home staffed by carers whose massive commitment cannot overcome their lack of professional education and training? Given the complexities of diagnosis, the limitations of mental health legislation and the ever-increasing range of treatment options, how will primary healthcare services suddenly develop the capacity to cope with the special needs of this group of citizens? That is the challenge for practitioners in the 21st century. The response will have to be sufficient to overcome today's shortfalls in service and to provide a more comprehensive and person-centred model of care in which individual needs give rise to more appropriate provision. The problems are not simply dictated by a person's mental state; they are more to do with society's capacity and willingness to respond to that state of mind when it belongs to the most marginalised people with the most complex needs in our society. Our concern should not be simply that GPs lack the understanding to provide for them, when evidently so few other practitioners do either. Our concern should be as much that the needs of people with learning disabilities and mental disorder have too few champions. Our concern should be that they still have too little political influence to challenge the bastions of modern society and too small a voice to be heard above the clamour and din of competing interests at the healthcare table. It is not simply about health and illness; it is about *valuing people who are not the same as you.*

REFERENCES

Bournewood [1998] 3 W.L.R. 107

Department of Health 1999a Facing the facts: learning disability services. A policy impact study of social and health services. The Stationery Office, London

Department of Health 1999b Once a day. NHSE/Department of Health, London

Department of Health 1999c Review of the Mental Health Act 1983. Report of the Expert Committee. The Stationery Office, London

Department of Health 1999d Mental health: national service frameworks. The Stationery Office, London

Department of Health 2001 Valuing people: a new strategy for learning disability for the 21st century (Cm 5086). The Stationery Office, London

Department of Health and Social Security 1972 Better services for the mentally handicapped. HMSO, London

Department of Health and Welsh Office 1959 Mental Health Act. HMSO, London

Department of Health and Welsh Office 1983 Mental Health Act. HMSO, London

Department of Health and Welsh Office 1999 Code of practice for Mental Health Act 1983. The Stationery Office, London

Gear J, Gates B, Wray J 2000 Towards understanding behaviour in behavioural distress: concepts and strategies. Baillière Tindall/Royal College of Nursing, London

Lord Chancellor's Department 1997 Who decides: making decisions on behalf of mentally incapacitated adults. The Stationery Office, London

Matthews D 1996 The OK health check. Fairfield, Preston

May, Baker 1977 A short guide to mental illness for the family doctor. May and Baker, Dagenham

Meins W 1995 Symptoms of major depression in mentally retarded adults. Journal of Intellectual Disability Research 39: 41–45

Moss S 1996 Validity of the schizophrenia diagnosis of the Psychiatric Assessment Schedule for Adults with Developmental Disability (Pas-Add). British Journal of Psychiatry 168: 359–367

Quigley A, Murray G C, McKenzie K, Elliot G 2001 Staff knowledge about symptoms of mental health problems in people with learning disabilities. Journal of Learning Disabilities 5(3): 235–243

Scottish Executive 2000 The same as you? A review of services for people with learning disabilities. The Stationery Office, Edinburgh

Thomas C L, Vardara D R, Egan E (eds) 1993 Tabers cyclopedic medical dictionary. Davis, Philadelphia, PA

Thomson M 1998 The problem of mental deficiency; eugenics, democracy and social policy in Britain, c. 1870–1959. Oxford University Press, Oxford

Turkistani I Y A 2000 Chemotherapy and other physical treatments. In: Gear J, Gates B, Wray J (eds) Towards understanding behaviour in behavioural distress: concepts and strategies. Baillière Tindall/Royal College of Nursing, London

Turner S, Moss S 1996 The health needs of adults with learning disabilities and the Health of the Nation Strategy. Journal of Intellectual Disability Research 40(5): 440–447

5 Ethics and research involving people with learning disabilities

Peter Eldridge

OVERVIEW

Research is first and foremost a process for developing or contributing to knowledge. Where research is conducted on living subjects, however, the advancement of knowledge pursued by research may sometimes conflict with their interests. It is the central concern of research ethics to resolve these conflicts.

The need for ethical guidelines for medical research on human beings was first highlighted following the revelation of the horrendous experiments carried out by Nazi medical scientists on human subjects during World War II. The Nuremberg Code (1947) was subsequently drawn up, implementing at an international level a code of ethics to govern research on human subjects, chief among these being the need for the subject's consent. In 1964, the Declaration of Helsinki was adopted by the World Medical Association, providing a more comprehensive set of guidelines. The importance of consent was again emphasised.

This chapter considers the analysis of benefit and burden in research, the issue of informed consent, particularly where consent may be difficult to ascertain, and the role of ethics committees to oversee research.

WEIGHING UP BENEFITS AND BURDENS OF RESEARCH

In conducting research that is ethical, it is necessary to consider whether the benefits of the research are likely to outweigh the burdens, and whether the distribution of these burdens is likely to be just and fair.

The value of a project

There are many reasons for conducting a piece of research. Sometimes conducting research is a vital component of completing a course of study; at other times it may be necessary in order to advance one's career. However, for medical research, these reasons are never enough by themselves; it is vital to pursue new and worthwhile information that is relevant, either directly or indirectly, to patient care. Moreover, there ought to be a reasonable expectation that this outcome will be attained. Box 5.1 describes a project involving individuals with learning disabilities that illustrates many of the important factors to consider in devising a research project.

| Box 5.1 | Principles guiding a research proposal |

Project value. A learning disabilities nurse, Dave, is studying for an MSc in Health Service Management and Research. As part of his dissertation he must conduct a research project, for which he has chosen to look at the relationship between moderate exercise and challenging behaviour. This is an important but under-researched topic in learning disabilities health care.

Project design. Dave has devised a protocol that is capable of providing increased knowledge in this area. On the advice of his supervisor he has increased the number of subjects in the study to ensure that the study is not 'underpowered' (i.e. producing insufficient data to yield significant results).

Choice of subjects. Dave will be recruiting people with learning disabilities to the project. Dave is aware that the learning disabilities clients in the Trust where he works are often used in research, but since his research should be of some benefit to participating clients, he does not want to exclude clients who are already research subjects in other projects. By contrast, one of Dave's colleagues is conducting non-therapeutic research in the same Trust to investigate the possibility of a genetic link with Asperger's syndrome. To prevent clients from being over-researched, an exclusion criteria will be participation in any other invasive research project over the past year.

Benefit versus burden. The benefits are twofold: those in the exercise arm of the study are expected to achieve some health gain, which would be of immediate therapeutic benefit, and the anticipated increase in medical knowledge should help many other learning disabled clients in the long term. The burdens are that the exercise may be physically and emotionally draining for subjects in the exercise arm, and for all subjects, including controls, participation may be of some inconvenience. Dave feels that these burdens are outweighed by the benefits, but will nonetheless take further steps to minimise them.

Minimising any burden. The exercise plan Dave has devised is essential to achieving his research aims and carries minimal risks, but it may nonetheless prove a physical and emotional burden. He has therefore chosen an outcome measurement that does not cause any more inconvenience: the effectiveness of exercise on reducing challenging behaviour will be evaluated using rating scales for measuring mental well-being, which can be completed on behalf of the subjects by the investigator team, rather than by using patient diaries.

In order for staff to develop research-based knowledge, it is important that they learn research skills. This, in turn, may lead to a large number of projects being undertaken by staff as part of their academic studies. Resource constraints, in particular a lack of time, may restrict the size of such studies, which may compromise the usefulness and the validity of generalising from the findings. If a medical research project is not intended to, or is unlikely to, make a contribution to medical knowledge, then its significance and value are highly questionable.

Within a climate of increased pressure to carry out research (whether to fulfil academic or professional requirements), it is important that this consideration is not overlooked.

Exploitation of subjects

The inequality in knowledge and vulnerability between investigators and subjects has the potential to lead to relationships that are exploitative (Beauchamp and Childress, 1994). Medical research must, therefore, not only be of benefit, it must be of sufficient benefit, either to the subject of research or to society in general, to outweigh any risks or inconvenience that the research may entail. This may include not just physical harm but also emotional or psychological distress. For instance, questionnaires and interviews, though physically uninvasive, may prove very demanding to subjects, depending on their content. Studies that explore personal experiences such as abuse, or the death of a loved one, may prove particularly stressful. People with learning disabilities may be especially susceptible to emotional and psychological upset.

Level of risk

It should be borne in mind that, even where it is necessary to achieve the research aims, the exposure of subjects to high levels of risk, particularly in research where the subjects themselves do not stand to receive any therapeutic benefit ('non-therapeutic' research), is likely to be limited by the law (Grubb, 1997).

The balance between risk and benefit must be considered for each project. An acceptable level of risk for investigation of the common cold will differ from that associated with a last resort cancer treatment. Individuals participating in research projects ought not to be subjected to any avoidable hazards, for no matter the benefits that the research may generate, they cannot be served by exposing subjects to risks superfluous to addressing the research question. Researchers should, therefore, act in such a way as to minimise the burdens placed on research subjects. To this end, adequate facilities for supervision and/or care must be provided before, during and after research.

Complexities that may be associated with research on certain patient groups, including those with learning disabilities, require even more careful supervision. People with learning disabilities may be especially susceptible to emotional and psychological trauma, creating a greater need for sensitivity on behalf of the researcher.

Obviously, human subjects ought not be used in research when the same increase in knowledge would be otherwise attainable. Where the advancement of medical knowledge does call for research on human subjects, it is important that the subject group is carefully considered. Is it essential to use a particular subject group? Recruitment of research subjects from a specific group must be justified to avoid unnecessarily shifting the burdens of research to certain subsections of society, particularly if they do not stand to share the benefits of that research. Identifying groups and predicting the distribution of burdens and benefits across them can be difficult, but certain lines may be drawn along socio-economic levels: between the healthy and the physically or psychologically unwell, the rich and the poor, the well educated and the poorly educated, the influential and the non-influential, the socially accepted and the socially marginalised, etc.

In recruiting subjects, researchers must fight a temptation to go to the most convenient source of supply, instead endeavouring to achieve a just recruitment process. While some valid research projects may require the use of individuals from particular subject groups, researchers must be aware of the dangers of over-researching these groups, especially when their minority status places them in high demand. This may be the case with people with learning disabilities.

Monetary recompense Certain subsections of society may be rendered vulnerable because of socio-economic factors. It is vital that researchers do not capitalise on this vulnerability. Intentionally or unintentionally, inducements offered for participation in research may exploit individuals whose circumstances render them particularly susceptible to this kind of incentive. Subjects may feel inclined to take unreasonable risks because of a lack of other viable options. For instance, if monetary inducements are offered, financial hardships may place undue pressure on individuals to participate in research they would otherwise reject.

Controls A final consideration is the provision of control or comparison subjects. Even if the aim of a piece of research is exceptionally laudable, its use and the contribution of its participants may be wasted if the project is not carefully planned to analyse any effect observed. Such a control group may be a similar group who receive no intervention, a historical group from medical records or a group receiving a different treatment. This aspect also needs ethical consideration.

INFORMED CONSENT Consent is the most important moral constraint that must be satisfied in conducting ethically sound medical research. It is important to recognise that, in both research and health-care practice, obtaining consent is much more than the mere satisfaction of a legal or social formality—it is a safeguard against exploitation or harm through fraud or duress. It is, therefore, imperative that consent be both freely given and appropriately informed. There are, however, certain complications involved in guaranteeing both these constituents of valid consent. While, generally speaking, every effort is made to shun active coercion, unintentional pressures placed on individuals to participate in research may be harder to avoid. These factors are discussed below and illustrated in Box 5.2.

Box 5.2	**Recruitment to a research project**

Project. A doctor working in the field of learning disabilities, Daisy, wants to take part in a national drug trial to test a new anti-epilepsy drug. While she is confident that the study is well designed, and that the outcome will inform future treatment of epilepsy that will benefit her patient group, she also wants to make sure that recruitment for this study is ethical.

Freely given consent. Daisy will be recruiting her own patients to this trial. Many of them trust her and consider her their friend. Although she will explain how the study may be of benefit to them, she must ensure that when she asks them for their consent, she makes it clear that this study is not an essential part of their care, and that her invitation to participate is as a researcher, and is not necessarily a clinical recommendation. She will emphasise that participation is voluntary, and that they will in no way be penalised if they refuse to take part.

Informed consent. Daisy will explain the whole research process to them: why the study is being done, how it is being conducted and what participation will involve (particularly what will be additional to their normal care). Daisy will take particular care to ensure that her patients understand that they will be taking part in a randomised, double-blind experiment involving a new drug, and that participation will offer a 50% chance of being given the new drug and a 50% chance of continuing to receive their current medication (though neither the subjects nor herself will know which).

Some of her patients will need to undergo an MRI (magnetic resonance imaging) scan and, although this is risk free, it can be noisy and may cause claustrophobia. Some of the study processes involve complex blood tests and an EEG (electroencephalograph). Rather than glossing over these procedures, Daisy will explain to her patients in simple terms what they involve.

Anonymity of results. Daisy will also reassure them that, although she hopes to publish the study, all of the study data will be anonymous, and that once the study is complete all the blood samples that she has collected will be destroyed.

In a separate project with clients from the Trust, involving tape-recorded interviews, anonymity was also an issue. Potential participants were informed who would have access to the tapes, how they would be analysed and how confidentiality and anonymity would be safeguarded.

Allowing time to consider. Since there is no reason for patients to enter the drug trial immediately, they can be given plenty of time to consider their decision. They are told that they do not have to give a reason if they choose not to participate, because this might place unnecessary pressure on them. They are also assured that once the study has started they may withdraw at any time. The potential participants will be provided with written information explaining all of the above information in clear terms. This cannot, however, be considered a substitute for a clear verbal explanation.

Ensuring consent is freely given Consent must involve an element of choice, which, in turn, requires that a range of available viable options be known from which to choose. Otherwise, decisions may be forced by the pressures of circumstance.

Fear of loss of care An individual's decision to participate in research may, for instance, be unduly influenced by virtue of an existing relationship with the researcher. Whether out of a certain misguided sense of duty, or because of some perceived threat to their standard of care should they refuse, people may feel obliged to cooperate if invited to take part in research conducted by a health-care worker responsible for their care. For example, a person invited to take part in a study by their GP could believe that a refusal would jeopardise their existing relationship, or perhaps even prejudice the service they receive. This may compromise the voluntary nature of any decision to take part. It must therefore be clearly articulated to prospective subjects that their participation is wholly voluntary, and that once research is underway they may pull out at any time. Moreover, they must be aware that refusal to participate, or withdrawal from the study, will incur no penalty.

Trust in a professional If a bond of professional trust already exists between the medical researcher and the people invited to participate in research, for example between doctors and their patients, then some individuals may defer to what they perceive to be their health-carer's better judgement regarding their care.

This pressure is perhaps most keenly felt in therapeutic research. A distinction is frequently made between therapeutic and non-therapeutic research, dating back to the Declaration of Helsinki. Whereas the purpose of non-therapeutic research is rarely the immediate benefit of the subject, it is commonly assumed that this is the purpose of therapeutic research. However, as discussed at the outset of this chapter, the primary goal of research is the advancement of knowledge and consequently it is seldom directly aimed at the immediate treatment of a patient's ills, even if it does involve some therapeutic intervention. Rather, research and therapy constitute dual aims of the intervention.

To acquire treatment Participation in research may sometimes be necessary in order to access particular forms of treatment; additionally, monitoring the effects of this treatment for research purposes may not adversely affect the patient. Nonetheless, research is almost always extra to, rather than a constituent of, therapy; consequently, it is rarely of necessity to the effective treatment of a patient. Patients who are unaware of this fact may misevaluate the advantages and disadvantages of their participation in research. Moreover, while there is no guarantee that participation in therapeutic research will benefit patients, anxiety and stress associated with illness may compromise the patient's capacity for rational decision making.

Therefore, when recruiting subjects to research studies, particularly therapeutic research studies, health-care researchers should take great care to distinguish between their advice as a carer and their requirements as a researcher.

Ability to give consent

People with learning disabilities may be particularly susceptible to the pressures outlined above since they are more likely to be dependent on their carers, not only for physical care but also for emotional support and guidance in decision making.

What is informed consent?

As discussed, consent must also be appropriately informed if it is to be considered valid. One must thus consider both the manner in which information is disclosed and its content. Ideally, a clear verbal explanation, with time to ask questions, should also be followed by written details and a period of time to reflect and maybe to form more questions. In recruiting people with learning disabilities, researchers must be particularly wary, as problems of understanding may be compounded.

Risks versus benefits

Individuals must be made aware of any risks or harms that might be posed to them by virtue of their participation in research. A study by Gerry Kent has revealed a marked divergence between the public's conception of the role of research ethics committees and that of the committee members (Kent, 1997). He suggests that potential subjects may view approval by an ethics committee as a guarantee that a research project poses no risks.

Risks and harms need not be restricted to physical hazards. Variations exist between different individuals in the weighing up of benefits and burdens, both physical and non-physical, not all of which might be considered rational. For instance, certain people might refuse to participate in otherwise relatively risk-free research on grounds peculiar to their own set of religious beliefs. Potential subjects of research should, therefore, be given ample information to allow them to form a decision in accordance with their personal values. This information should include at least the nature, duration and purpose of the experiment, as well as the method by which it is to be conducted. The presence of randomisation or blinding also warrants disclosure on these grounds.

Access to results

It is also important that potential subjects are informed who will have access to personal information about them and the research findings, as well as how confidentiality and anonymity will be assured.

The importance of providing them with this information is twofold. First, they may have valid concerns regarding potential invasions of privacy. Second, the disclosure of certain information may carry far-reaching effects for participants, such as social stigmatisation or an adverse affect on life or health insurance. How information about a subject's genetic predisposition to certain diseases or their human immunodeficiency (HIV) status is stored, for instance, may be of particular concern.

Even information outside the immediate scope of the research project may nonetheless be of relevance to subjects. They should, for instance, be told what will happen to any tissue samples that they donate for the project—whether they will be destroyed once the study is over or stored for teaching purposes or future research projects.

Explanation of the programme

Many individuals invited to participate in research will find the medical jargon frequently used in describing research projects incomprehensible. Even words commonly used by the lay population may be inaccurately understood, such as 'CAT scan', 'placebo' and 'haemorrhoids'. Some non-clinical words, such as 'standard', may find a very different usage in a clinical context. Consequently, it is important that the disclosure of information suits the potential subject's level of understanding, although, of course, a lack of medical knowledge in the potential subject is no excuse for withholding relevant information or distorting the facts (e.g. by understating certain risks involved).

An explanation given in simple language may still be muddled or confusing. In order to minimise further the potential for misunderstanding, information must be communicated as clearly as possible.

Ongoing aspects of consent

Obtaining consent ought not to be viewed as a 'gateway event', after which a person's willingness and understanding may be taken for granted. Rather, it should be understood as an ongoing process that will continue for the duration of the subject's involvement. A person's willingness to participate, and understanding of what it is that they are participating in, should be checked periodically, particularly if the researcher has reason to believe that one of these two essential elements of valid consent may have changed (e.g. if the subject suggests that they are reluctant to continue in the project, or that they no longer understand some aspect of the research project pertinent to their decision to participate).

RESEARCH IN THOSE UNABLE TO GIVE INFORMED CONSENT

A great many people with learning disabilities suffer from communication difficulties. Although this may make it difficult to communicate information to them regarding their circumstances, the options available to them, and the likely outcomes of pursuing any one of these options, it does not make it impossible. These individuals may, therefore, still be capable of giving informed consent to participate in research projects.

Individuals who are capable of giving informed consent may not be able to do so on all occasions. Some, because of age, illness or disability, may be incapable of fully understanding their circumstances, regardless of how this information may be presented to them. In such situations, they may be incapable of making suitably informed decisions regarding what course of action they wish to take and how they wish to be treated; this situation can occur with all potential participants, not just those who have learning disabilities.

The capacity to make informed decisions is often context dependent. Although some may lose, or simply never even gain, this capacity, others may possess it some but not all of the time. Much will depend on the complexity of the situation they are presented with. Although they may find it hard or impossible to comprehend certain situations, this does not necessarily mean that they are incapable of comprehending any situation whatsoever. Capacity will also be subject to variations in mental state, for example whether the individual is unconscious, distressed or confused.

The mere presence of learning disability, mental disorder or obstacles to the communication of information should never in itself be considered sufficient to demonstrate that an individual is incapable of ever giving informed consent. Nontheless, there will be some individuals for whom giving informed consent may be an impossibility.

Legal and ethical dimensions

In any discussion of research conducted on people who are incapable of consenting to participation, it is important to consider both the legal and ethical dimensions. Though there are similarities between the legal and ethical requirements concerning how people who cannot make informed decisions should be treated, it should be borne in mind that there are also differences: what is ethical is not always legal, and vice versa.

If the value of self-determination and freedom from external interference (whether physical or psychological) is to be recognised and respected, then it is important to gain consent from an individual before things are done to them, particularly if one intends to interact with them physically. Under English law, individuals have the right to decide what is done to their own body. It is, therefore, unlawful, whatever one's intention, to touch or otherwise interfere with another person's body without their permission. Where such contact is particularly invasive, it may be considered a case of battery. Ethically, there are circumstances in which non-consensual bodily contact may be considered acceptable, and many of these are reflected in law. For example, the inevitable contact of everyday social interaction is not considered illegal, nor is it necessarily illegal to restrain a person physically whose behaviour constitutes a threat to themselves or others.

Proxy consent   A degree of bodily contact will at times be necessary to promote or protect the well-being of individuals who are either temporarily or permanently incapable of giving consent. Therefore, proxy consent—that is, consent given on a person's behalf—to physical or psychological interference can be considered a morally acceptable substitute where such interference is necessary to preserve or further their interests. Failing to administer treatment to a sick person on the grounds that it is not possible to obtain their consent may sometimes result in a decline in their health, or even in their death. Consequently, although in health-care practice the wishes of the individual are usually considered paramount, in certain circumstances consent by proxy will be acceptable.

Under English law, a suitable person such as a parent or legal guardian may consent on a minor's behalf; however, no one may consent for medical treatment or for participation in medical research on behalf of an adult, even if that adult is incapable of giving consent themselves. Nonetheless, the law recognises the importance of being able to provide health care to such adults, and, therefore, it is legal for emergency treatment and, more recently, for any treatment that is in the best interests of a patient (i.e. necessary to preserve life or improve/prevent a deterioration in physical or mental health; see Re F [1990: sterilisation for a mentally ill patient]) to be administered to adults who cannot consent.

It is apparent, then, that a distinction exists under English law between obtaining proxy consent to treatment for an incapable person and treating an incapable person on the grounds that it is in their best interests. Although only the latter process is considered legal for adults, there is little to distinguish these arrangements from one another. Both involve treating a patient who cannot consent to treatment on the grounds that another person, whose opinion it is deemed suitable to consult, sanctions this behaviour, and whose authority, in turn, stems from the fact that they act in the patient's interests. Subtle legal differences may be implied as to whom it is deemed appropriate to consult, in what circumstances they may be consulted and what authority their decisions carry, but ethically, these two arrangements are equivalent.

Proxy consent for research The Declaration of Helsinki allows that permission may be obtained from a responsible relative or legal guardian for an individual to participate in research if that individual is incapable of giving informed consent, whether because of physical or mental incapacity or legal status as a minor, and if this is in accordance with national legislation (Faulder, 1985). However, exactly when incapable individuals may be allowed to participate in research is rather unclear under English law.

Participation in therapeutic research will sometimes be in the best interests of an incapable person, offering many of the same benefits as treatment that is not research related. The moral justification for proxy consent may thus be extended to some cases of therapeutic research, and for children at least, this is acceptable under English law. Moreover, since the law permits incapable adults to be treated, provided that such treatment is necessary to protect and further their best interests, it seems only sensible to assume that where such treatment forms part of a research project, this will likewise be acceptable in law (although this is by no means explicit under current legislation).

At first glance, non-therapeutic research would not appear to be in the best interests of subjects unable to make an informed decision to participate. However, interests need not be restricted simply to physical well-being but may also include emotional and psychological satisfaction. The courts allowed an incapable adult to act as a bone marrow donor to her seriously ill sister on the grounds that the emotional benefit she gained by helping generated a sufficiently strong interest to outweigh the relatively small physical risks she faced (see Re Y, 1996). It is possible that the satisfaction of altruistic intentions might similarly render participation in non-therapeutic research in the best interests of incapable individuals, and therefore morally acceptable, provided that the risks to the subject are minimal.

Substituted judgement While individuals incapable of making informed decisions may have preferences concerning how they are treated, as discussed, many have difficulty communicating these. In such cases, it can be helpful for those who know them to estimate what these preferences might be, in other words attempting to answer 'what would they want?'. This process is known as 'substituted judgement'. Consideration may be given not only to the satisfaction of incapable individuals' current preferences but also to the fulfilment of preferences that they may have expressed whilst deemed capable. Substituted judgement can, therefore, be used to ascertain what an individual's preferences are, were and in all likelihood would otherwise have been, and thus to identify their interests. Substituted judgement will often be most accurately given from, or in consultation with, a person's relatives.

It follows, then, that even if participation in a non-therapeutic research project does not constitute a necessary part of an incapable individual's treatment, it may nonetheless be in their interests and substituted judgement would support participation (see Box 5.3). It does not follow, however, that these wider, non treatment-related interests would be acceptable grounds under English law to allow the participation of incapable adults in non-therapeutic research. Indeed, it is quite possible that non-therapeutic research on incapable adults, even with the agreement of their relatives, is illegal, particularly where it involves some physical contact.

Box 5.3	**Research where clear consent is not possible**

Project. Wayne is a researcher who wants to compare the care provided by learning disabilities specialists with that of mental health specialists. The comparison would be based on interviews with carers, service users and their families, as well as an examination of the subjects' personal health records.

For the sample to be representative, it must include a broad range of people with learning disabilities and, given the increased vulnerability of those with severe learning disabilities, it is important that this group be included. Therefore some of the clients that Wayne needs to study may be incapable of giving informed consent.

By contrast, a separate project involving clients from the same Trust had initially considered including clients unable to consent, but was changed because the research question could be answered without recruiting such subjects.

Benefits and burdens. The research does not appear to be in the best immediate interests of the clients. It in no way forms part of their care nor is it likely to fulfil any specific emotional desires. The research is, however, necessary to bring about improvements in the standard of learning disabilities health care. It is likely to be of particular importance for incapable clients with learning disabilities, although it may not necessarily be of benefit to the individuals involved in the study. Moreover, if the research does not go ahead, it may have adverse repercussions for many people with learning disabilities. The interviews would not be very probing and the researcher has experience working with people with learning disabilities, so it is unlikely to cause the subjects distress.

Grounds for proceeding without consent. On balance, Wayne believes there is a strong case for proceeding with the research without informed consent from all the clients (though, of course, he will make every effort to inform them as much as possible, and to make doubly sure that they do not have any objections). Moreover, where possible the relatives will be informed about the study so that they can give their opinion. They may be able to provide an insight into whether their relative would normally be willing to help out in this manner by taking part in research or whether the research is likely to be against their best interests (they may, for instance, be very private people, or nervous around strangers).

Of course, some non-therapeutic research projects will never be in the interests of incapable subjects, no matter how widely interests are defined. Since the primary duty of a person responsible for an incapable individual is to ensure that that individual's interests are served, and the decisions they make on their behalf would appear to be authoritative only in so far as they accord with this principle, the moral justification for proxy consent is absent where such projects are concerned. Curiously, however, because of the way in which proxy consent applies to children under English law, parents are still allowed to give proxy consent for their children to participate in research that is not in their interests, providing that it is not *against* their interests, for example if there is minimal risk or inconvenience involved (e.g. questionnaires).

An alternative moral argument for the recruitment of incapable subjects to research projects that do not lie in their interest is that the benefits of such research justify the burdens imposed on the subjects. If the potential benefits of research are sufficiently large, and the risks and inconvenience posed to participants are sufficiently small, then this may outweigh the subjects' entitlement to self-determination and freedom from external interference. Indeed, it may be considered unethical *not* to proceed. It should be noted that this argument, which may be used alone or in combination with the 'best interests' argument in building the moral case in favour of allowing incapable patients to participate in research, is not recognised in English law.

In discussions concerning the legal and ethical dimensions of research on incapable individuals, it is generally agreed that no one may be recruited into a study if, either through their words or their actions, they object or appear to object, even if they are deemed incapable in this instance of making an informed decision. However, though it is clear that by ignoring such an objection one would be acting against that person's wishes, it does not thereby follow that one would be acting against their interests. Administration of medical treatment to promote or protect an individual's health, but to which that individual, incapable of fully comprehending his or her circumstances, objects, may nonetheless be in their interests. Such behaviour is ethical, but it is unclear whether it would be considered legal under English law, nor, if it was, whether this might extend to some therapeutic research.

In treating or conducting research on incapable individuals, it is customary to inform and seek the approval of their relatives. Relatives' opinions may be valuable in evaluating whether such behaviour is ethical, particularly where they offer some new perspective on a patient's desires and preferences. Moreover, involvement in the decision-making process may serve to reassure relatives and exclusion may alienate them. While such consultation is considered good practice, it is by no means obvious that it is necessary in law; additionally, where incapable adults are concerned, it will not in itself be sufficient to render either treatment or research legal.

RESEARCH ETHICS COMMITTEES

All research in the UK involving people by virtue of their past or present status as NHS patients or users, or involving NHS staff (either as researchers or research subjects), must be subjected to ethical review by an NHS research ethics committee. The purpose of research ethics committees is to ensure that proposed research projects will not expose the subjects involved to unacceptable risks or practices, and that potential subjects will be able to make an informed decision as to whether or not to participate in approved studies. Committees also bear the wider responsibility of promoting the public interest by helping to ensure that valid and relevant research is carried out.

Whilst ethical analysis is a priority, the scientific merit of a proposed research project does, of course, have ethical implications, as described above. Research indicates that the researchers themselves do not consider an evaluation of methodological soundness to be as important a role for the local research ethics committees as committee members do, which may partly explain the annoyance of researchers when their research projects are rejected on methodological grounds (Kent, 1997).

A number of studies have drawn attention to the differences and inconsistencies that exist between the judgements of local research ethics committees. Hotopf, Wessely and Noah (1995) sent the same proposal to six local research ethics committees to assess the degree of agreement between them. All but one committee demanded significant changes, yet none asked for the same changes. Numerous studies echo these findings (Ahmed and Nicholson, 1996; Gilbert, Fulford and Parker, 1989; Harries et al., 1994; Hoptopf et al., 1995; Kent, 1997; Redshaw, Harris and Baurn, 1996; While, 1995).

Approval from a research ethics committee

Certain groups, such as people with learning disabilities, may be particularly vulnerable to exploitation, be it deliberate or unintentional. It is, therefore, important that research on such vulnerable groups is thoroughly reviewed, and it is likely that such research will be subjected to close scrutiny.

However, the fact that different research ethics committees may often view the same project differently makes it very hard to provide hard and fast guidelines for gaining approval for a project. While it is important to plan a research study that is ethical, this in itself may not be sufficient to guarantee approval by a research ethics committee.

Unless the study is fully and clearly explained in the application, it may be misunderstood by the committee.

The following pointers should make life easier for researchers and research ethics committees:

- Applications should be easy to understand. Research applications that presume an understanding of the field concerned may be hard to understand for health care professional members of research ethics committees, let alone the lay members.
- Applications should be transparently methodologically sound. As explained above, this is a legitimate concern of a research ethics committee.
- Applications should be transparently ethically sound. If the research is likely to be ethically problematic (for instance, if it is particularly invasive or if it involves people incapable of giving informed consent), it should be evident that these issues have been recognised and, more importantly, addressed.
- Applications should be complete! NHS research ethics committees provide guidelines for submitting applications for review, and these should be read and followed to the letter. Failing to provide required information (such as proposed recruitment figures, study documents or even signatures) can waste considerable time and is easily avoidable.
- It can pay dividends to communicate effectively with the research ethics committee. If any aspect of the application process is unclear, asking questions can save valuable time and effort.

CONCLUSIONS Research should never be undertaken until the ethical implications have been considered. The potential benefits of research should always be carefully weighed against the potential burdens, and whilst this may sometimes be a very fine balancing act, familiarity with the ethical concerns described in this chapter should serve to clarify and facilitate this process.

REFERENCES Ahmed A, Nicholson K 1996 Delays and diversity in the practice of local research ethics committees. Journal of Medical Ethics 22: 263–266

Beauchamp, T L, Childress J F 1994 Principles of biomedical ethics, 4th edn. Oxford University Press, Oxford

Faulder C 1985 Whose body is it? The troubling issue of informed consent. Virago, London

Gilbert C, Fulford K, Parker C 1989 Diversity of the practice of district ethics committees. British Medical Journal 299: 1437–1439

Grubb A 1997 The law relating to consent. In: Foster C (ed) Manual for research ethics committees, 5th edn. King's College, London, pII, point 17–22

Harries H, Fentem P, Tuxworth W, Hoinville G 1994 Local research ethics committees. Journal of the Royal College of Physicians of London 28: 150–154

Hoptopf M, Wessely S, Noah N 1995 Are ethical committees reliable? Journal of the Royal Society of Medicine 88: 31–33

Kent G 1997 The views of members of local research ethics committees, researchers and members of the public towards the roles and functions of LRECs. Journal of Medical Ethics 23: 186–190

Re F (sterilisation for a mentally ill patient) [1990] 2 AC 112

Re Y (mental incapacity: bone marrow transplant) [1996] 2 FLR 787

Redshaw M E, Harris A, Baurn J D 1996 Research ethics committee audit: differences between committees. Journal of Medical Ethics 22: 78–82

While A E 1995 Ethics committees: impediments to research or guardians of ethical standards? British Medical Journal 311: 661

6

Bereavement and loss

Sue Read

OVERVIEW The broad aim of this chapter is to introduce the key issues involved when supporting the individual who has a learning disability experiencing loss within a context of death and dying, specifically from the perspective of learning disability nursing. The concept of loss and typical grief responses are discussed and related to the issues and challenges often posed by this client group when experiencing loss, death or bereavement. Support strategies and current developments are explored in differing loss contexts.

Although the focus of the chapter is around loss and bereavement, the issues posed by individuals with a learning disability when faced with an illness requiring palliative care will also be introduced. Since this is a relatively new area of practice development, it contains many practice-related issues and will ultimately involve learning disability nurses. Specifically, the aims of this chapter are to:

- define the concept of loss
- identify and acknowledge the potential impact of loss on the individual
- identify the challenges often associated with supporting loss in the individual with a learning disability
- explore the needs of the person with a learning disability within palliative care
- clarify the role of the nurse in providing proactive and reactive support
- develop positive practice.

This chapter concludes by offering a checklist for positive practice, which is offered as a guide to evaluate current service and practice and to identify the need for future developments within this sensitive and often complex area.

INTRODUCTION Loss means different things to different people and occurs in a variety of differing contexts: 'I thought that it sometimes seems as if all our lives we are trying to cope with loss—either the fear of it, or the memory of it, or its raw immediate presence' (Oswin, 2000, p 21). Weston et al. (1998, p 4) described loss specifically thus: 'To lose something or somebody is to be deprived of, and separated from, a presence, often taken for granted, around which or whom we have organised our lives'; while Machin (1998) described loss simplistically as losing what we want to keep. A group of eight people with learning disability described loss from within a more broad-based context (Read et al., 2000):

- loss of self, confusion, frustration at not understanding what others were saying and not being given the opportunity to communicate their own thoughts, feelings and emotions
- losing control over important life decisions, feeling they had no choice about where or with whom they were going to live after a close relative had died.

Clearly, loss is not just about death but may encompass a whole range of experiences, often related to change. Life often involves change, and all life changes have an element of loss (Fisher and Warman, 1990). For people with learning disabilities, change has been an important, consistent feature over the years as national policy developments (such as *Caring for people*, Department of Health, 1989) supported huge changes in their lives through community integration policies. The gradual relocation of many people with learning disabilities over the years has meant enormous changes in lifestyles as individuals have had to adjust and adapt to small, community-based living opportunities in contrast to the large, segregated facilities of their past.

What is also clear is that individuals generally may respond to loss in a variety of ways and develop personal coping strategies, which are established over time through previous (positive and negative) experiences (Machin, 1998). For many people with a learning disability, such coping mechanisms may be very limited and often can be non-existent, as historically such people have not been afforded appropriate support when experiencing a loss in their lives and have not been actively involved in the sad business of death and dying. Indeed, for many people with a learning disability, loss has not even been acknowledged as being an important feature in their lives, or as a factor affecting their lifestyles. Fortunately, many professional groups are now becoming aware of the loss and bereavement needs of this client group and are attempting to address such hidden needs in a proactive, sensitive and supportive way.

LOSS
The impact of loss

Death is the most difficult of losses to accommodate (Holmes and Rahe, 1967), and how we respond to death is often described as grief.

Table 6.1
Grief responses

Type of response	Typical features
Emotional	Sadness, anger, guilt, self reproach, anxiety, loneliness, fatigue, helplessness, shock, yearning, relief, numbness
Physical	Hollowness in the stomach, tightness in the chest, tightness in the throat, oversensitivity to noise, a sense of depersonalisation, breathlessness, weakness in the muscles, lack of energy, dry mouth
Behavioural	Sleep disturbance, appetite disturbance, absentmindedness, social withdrawal, dreaming, searching, crying, sighing, restless over-activity, visiting old haunts
Psychological	Disbelief, confusion, preoccupation, sense of presence, hallucinations

After Worden (1991, pp 222–230).

Table 6.2
Grief theories

Author	Tasks or phases passed through in grief
Lindemann (1944)	Shock, acute mourning, resolution
Kubler-Ross (1969)	Denial, anger, guilt, depression
Parkes (1975)	Numbness, searching/pining, depression, recovery
Bowlby (1996)	Numbing, searching, disorganisation and despair, adjustment
Worden (1991)	Accept the reality of the loss, work through the pain of grief, adjust to life without the missing person or object, re-investment in new life

After Cooley (1992).

Grief is a response to loss that can have social, psychological, behavioural, physical or emotional facets (according to Worden, 1991). Table 6.1 lists some of the typical responses.

Although each individual responds to loss in a personal and unique way, numerous authors and researchers over recent years have identified common reactions within tasks or phases displayed by grieving individuals; these have been incorporated into theories of grief (Table 6.2). More recent models include the dual process model by Stroebe and Schutt (1996), which depicts bereaved people as oscillating between either loss-focussed (grief) work or restoration-focussed (moving on with life) orientations. Klass et al. (1996) focussed upon the importance of maintaining a relationship with the deceased, which may change over time but may last indefinitely.

Clearly, what all these models support is the need for the bereaved individual to feel able to explore personal responses to loss before moving on with life as the loss is accommodated into the life of the living (Worden, 1991). Each model has something to contribute to our understanding of healthy grief work.

Sometimes, however, events or circumstances surrounding the death may serve to make it more difficult or complex, resulting in what

Fisher and Warman (1990) described as either delayed grief (for example inhibited, suppressed or postponed grief) or chronic grief (where the grief remains excessive in duration or exaggerated). Circumstances that may serve to complicate grief reactions include sudden death, the nature of the death (for example murder or suicide), multiple deaths, not being able to say goodbye, multiple losses and the age of the dead person (for example, a child's death is perceived as being very difficult to cope with). For people with learning disabilities, factors that serve to complicate their grief work centre largely around the challenges involved in communicating and working with this group, which are identified later in this chapter.

Bereavement models can help professionals to understand how bereaved individuals might be feeling and can support bereavement counsellors actively in their work of grief facilitation. A meaningful model or framework for support of those with a learning disability needs to be identified. To do this, we need to explore the relationship between bereavement generally and learning disability specifically.

Loss and learning disability

Oswin (2000, p 31) stated, '… despite all the advances made in changing attitudes towards people with learning difficulties, it appears that in the area of loss and bereavement they are still not receiving enough consideration, nor the appropriate support they require…'. A steady trickle of literature over recent years has helped to raise awareness of the effects of bereavement in the learning disabled and to identify the particular needs and associated challenges. The impact of bereavement on behaviour in this group was noted initially by Emerson (1977), who related grief to emotional and management difficulties. Later, Conboy-Hill (1992) cited grief as a major contributor to numerous behavioural problems, including self-injury, loss of skills, anorexia and aggression. The predisposition of bereavement leading to mental health problems was identified by both Ray (1978) and Bimh and Elliot (1982). More recently, Bonell-Pascual et al. (2000) identified a small increase in the measures of aberrant behaviour of 50 bereaved people with learning disabilities over a 5-year follow-up study.

There have also been many case illustrations which demonstrated that people with learning disabilities do grieve (Clarke and Read, 1998; Elliot, 1995; Kitching, 1987), do experience loss (Service et al., 1999) and often respond to such experiences in a very profound way. A workshop experience on loss and change for adults with learning disabilities (Read et al., 2000) explicitly identified the normality of grief expressed by the eight participants, describing physical responses (crying and shaking), psychological responses (such as confusion, suppressing feelings, missing and thinking about the deceased) and profound sadness.

Clearly, people with learning disabilities are affected when their loved ones die. According to Bonell-Pascual et al. (2000), 'the response to bereavement by adults with learning disability is similar in type, though not in expression, to that of the general population'. As the primary carers for many people with learning disability, learning disability nurses will have a pivotal role in supporting them with their grief, which includes identifying the particular challenges involved in this process.

Considering the challenges of loss

Dealing with death is never easy as it may confront many potential personal issues within the helper. Worden (1991, pp 133–134) suggested that working with death and dying generally affects individuals in three specific ways: it makes us painfully aware of our own loses, it makes us aware of our potential losses and it makes us aware of our own pending mortality.

Feelings about death is a very taboo and private subject, which many individuals may prefer to keep to themselves. Society generally contains a variety of death-denying cultures, as if to pretend that death itself is an event that either will not happen or does not pose problems. Consequently, there may be many challenges presenting to the professional carers of people with learning disability as they seek to overcome a host of personal, social, practical and historical barriers to offering sensitive and meaningful support at such a difficult time. Some of these challenges may relate to the nature of the learning disability itself while others relate to individual or societal belief systems often associated with learning disability. Kloeppel and Hollins (1989) coined the phrase 'Double handicap: retardation and death in the family' in recognition of the potential difficulties involved in dealing with both death and disability.

Emerson (1977) described a variety of responses when loss occurred in the lives of people with learning disabilities:

- professional or family carers either denied the event or trivialised it
- professionals, family or peers gave inappropriate responses to the individual
- family or professional carers did not allow or facilitate any emotional response from the individual
- the bereaved individual was not given adequate time to adjust to the changes that were consequential to the loss.

Crick (1988) suggested that the usual professional response when a person with a learning disability experienced a bereavement was either chemotherapy or behaviour therapy—both of which address the presenting symptoms but do not address the cause. Such responses are still prevalent, and Oswin (2000) suggested that a major reason for this is that carers (both personal and professional) are often afraid to explore other people's grief for fear of getting upset or because they are unsure about how to handle the situation. Oswin (2000, pp 33–35) goes on to describe how people with learning disabilities are often given confusing or mixed messages about death:

- They may be given peculiar ideas about the death, especially when those around them are using euphemisms about the death (for example, 'gone to sleep' 'gone away' or 'kicked the bucket').
- The individual might want to repeat verbally what has happened time and time again in an attempt to understand it, and find that carers prefer them to forget about it and be happy.
- They are often not told about a death because 'they won't understand' or might react badly.
- Some individuals might be told that 'they won't be visited anymore' with no concrete explanation as to why this may be so.

The media also offers confusing messages about death; for example, characters on the television often die and are then magically reconstructed in a different role on a different channel. To the person who has difficulty making sense of abstract concepts, death is portrayed as being reversible and not permanent. This can undo the very essence of what we try to reinforce (and may struggle to achieve) with people with a learning disability: understanding the finality of death and its inherent consequences.

Carers may decide not to tell the individual about a death for a number of reasons. They may believe that the person with a learning disability lacks the cognitive ability to comprehend what is being said to them, or may not understand the concept of death. They may simply be afraid of upsetting the individual by sharing or involving them in such difficult issues. Individuals who have challenging behaviours or additional mental health problems are even less likely to be told about the death of their loved ones for fear of precipitating anticipated challenging reactions.

Additionally, the more profound or complex the disability, the less likely the individual is to be actively involved and supported with a bereavement, largely because of anticipated communication challenges and their poor cognition, and, possibly, because of the narrow-minded attitudes of those caring for them.

Such prevailing, negative attitudes may include overprotectiveness, often caused by lack of knowledge and understanding but resulting in an unhealthy ignorance about dealing with death and bereavement. Specific challenges in relation to addressing the bereavement needs of this client group, from both the individual and the carer's perspective, can be summarised:

- emphatically bad attitudes (Oswin, 2000)
- disbelief that people with learning disabilities can grieve

- low expectations (Kitching, 1987)
- general cultural and societal taboos around both death and disability
- complexity of cognitive ability, limited attention span and limited emotional vocabulary (Conboy-Hill, 1992)
- lack of appropriate specialist education, training and supervision (Read, 1996)
- ways in which death is conceptualised
- treating the symptoms rather than addressing the cause (Crick, 1988)
- disempowerment
- lack of involvement or participation in death rituals
- lack of education/exploration of loss and bereavement
- lack of history and heritage
- confusing messages surrounding death generally.

Such responses articulate what Doka (1989) went on later to describe as disenfranchised grief, which he identified as 'the grief that persons experience when they incur a loss that is not or cannot be openly acknowledged, publicly mourned or socially supported'. Doka goes on to identify the three features of disenfranchised grief as:

- having the grief not recognised
- having the relationship not recognised
- having the griever not recognised.

Historically, people with learning disability have often not been informed of the death of their loved ones; there has been little (if any) recognition of the importance of relationships (either distant or close) and the individual has often been excluded from participating in the planning of the funeral arrangements and other associated rituals (for example choosing the flowers, selecting the hymns and visiting the Chapel of Rest) surrounding the death, as Jean's story (Box 6.1) illustrates.

Box 6.1	A delayed response to death: Jean's story

Jean was 62 years of age when she started to exhibit changes in her behaviour that were both socially unacceptable and totally out of character. Jean lost the many skills acquired over the years, became withdrawn and antisocial. She had had good communication skills, could read and write and used a wheelchair to get around. 7 years previously, her sister had died of cancer. Jean had nursed her sister (who also had a learning disability) and was with her when she eventually died. Jean had not attended the funeral, had no photographs of her sister, had no death certificate and did not even know where she was buried. She had never been to the graveside.

Because of the nature and circumstances of the death (a difficult death, no concrete memories, non-attendance at the funeral), Jean was referred to a bereavement counsellor for specific counselling and support.

Such disenfranchising responses may be perceived as paternalistic reactions; these may, in fairness, be incidental rather than deliberate, often in the effort to protect the individual who has a learning disability from the pain of grief. Unfortunately, experiencing the pain of grief is an important feature of accepting, responding to and accommodating the loss, and such disenfranchising responses serve to create additional problems while minimising any available support for the bereaved individual.

These responses serve to deny the reality and offer no positive affirmation or acknowledgement of the death to the bereaved individual. They also exclude the individual from experiencing the potential range of associated feelings and responses in healthy grief work at the time when other friends and relatives may be grieving.

Jean's story (Box 6.1) is a typical example of the bereavement experiences of people with learning disabilities. Jean may have been excluded from the funeral for a host of reasons (for example, limited accessibility to the church, she did not want to go, she was not asked if she wanted to go, staffing numbers meant no one could take her). However, not attending the funeral, combined with having no concrete or tangible memories (no photographs) and not having visited the graveside, has not afforded Jean any opportunity to see where her sister went to and does not affirm that she will not return. As Oswin (2000, p 35) states: 'An inability to recognise the person's grief will make them lonely at the very time that they need other people, love and friendship. They not only need their grief recognised, they also need permission to grieve . . .'. Giving permission to respond to loss is an important factor in the support for the bereaved individual. Jean's story will be revisited later, in an effort to explore positive approaches to her loss.

The challenges previously identified underpin any positive responses to people with learning disability who are suffering a loss. Clearly any loss and bereavement work to support this client group should initially be based around trying to prevent, minimise or address such disenfranchising effects, by addressing these identified challenges.

RECOGNISING ILL-HEALTH IN THOSE WITH A LEARNING DISABILITY

Similar challenges to those described in bereavement can also be identified when supporting the individual who has a palliative illness or may be personally facing a life-threatening illness. According to *The health of the nation* (Department of Health, 1995), 'People with learning disabilities should have access to all general health services, including health promotion and health education, and primary and secondary health care with appropriate additional support to meet those needs'.

However, such people often have additional health-care needs that may go unnoticed, and consequently untreated, and may have illnesses that remain undiagnosed until well advanced and hence too established to respond to active treatment (Tuffrey-Wijne, 1997). Positive routine, regular health promotion and access to screening programmes will be imperative for the early detection of illness for this client group. Documents such as those developed by the NHS Cancer Screening Programmes (2000) promoting good practice in breast and cervical screening for women with learning disabilities are a welcome and much needed development for professional carers and individuals alike.

Recognition of ill-health may be more difficult amongst people with learning disability because:

- the symptoms may not be easily identified, recognised or acknowledged
- the seriousness of the illness may be ignored or trivialised
- families and carers may not have the necessary skills or knowledge to support the individual with a learning disability in obtaining appropriate treatment or in the maintenance of health-related behaviour (Howells, 1997)
- individuals themselves may not know that anything is wrong (Keenan and McIntosh, 2000)
- individuals may have difficulties in communicating their discomfort or experience of severe pain (Keenan and McIntosh, 2000)
- individuals may be treated by some health and social care professionals as passive recipients (Keenan and McIntosh, 2000)
- poor communication channels may exist between individuals/organisations/professional disciplines.

PALLIATIVE CARE AND LEARNING DISABILITY

A developing area of concern from a primary care perspective is palliative care for the person who has a learning disability. The World Health Organization (1990) defined palliative care as 'The active total care of patients whose disease is not responsive to curative treatment. Control of pain, of other symptoms, and of psychological, social and spiritual problems, is paramount. The goal of palliative care is achievement of the best quality of life for patients and their families.' Consequently, palliative care is seen as incorporating any illness that does not currently have a cure and so does not just involve cancer-related illness. There is no reason to assume that people with learning disabilities will not experience the range of palliative care illnesses that other non-disabled individuals experience, and there are many examples of this in practice (for example, Bycroft, 1994). Palliative care may touch people with learning disability in three specific ways:

- when individuals themselves have a palliative illness
- when one of their family or friends has a palliative illness
- when their primary carer has a palliative illness.

Many years ago, when an individual with a learning disability experienced a palliative illness, this was treated within the auspices of the institution. With the implementation of community care initiatives, such individuals are now experiencing both palliative and terminal illnesses within the community setting. This means that people with learning disability are having to use generic primary care services, and there is evidence to suggest that such services are not adequately prepared to deal with those who have the combined needs of learning disability and palliative care (Lindop and Read, 2000). Although Nightingale et al. (1998) suggested that 'people with learning disability are no more poorly served than their local communities in general', this was from a primary care, not a palliative care, perspective.

Communication in palliative care

Good communication is the key to effective palliative care, whether communicating difficult news, diagnosis, prognosis or explaining symptom control and management. According to Kerr et al. (1996), over 50% of people with learning disabilities present with communication impairment. Such impairments can involve hearing impairment and/or speech and language disorders; these can all affect cognitive functioning and social interaction. Some individuals might use an alternative communication system, such as British Sign Language, which may not have the sophistication or the variety of symbols or gestures needed to communicate about death, dying or bereavement in a sensitive and meaningful way. From a palliative care perspective, such communication impairment might affect:

- the individual's ability to express emotion
- carer's ability to identify and address ill-health
- the ability of different professionals to respond to ill-health
- access to appropriate preventative screening opportunities
- the individual's ability to understand abstract concepts (such as death or loss)
- behaviour, precipitating tactile defence
- the individual's understanding of the concepts of loss, death or dying
- the individual's ability to receive, understand and respond to difficult news
- social interaction and interpersonal functioning

- the establishment and development of quality relationships
- the carer's ability to measure, monitor and evaluate pain and symptom management
- the individual's ability to ask questions
- the individual's autonomy
- the individual's right to be told (and receive) the truth.

Such communication challenges can be addressed in a number of ways by professionals (Read, 1998):

- allow an individual time to inspect/digest information, verbally or visually
- use visual stimuli such as books, pictures, photographs, together with short, simple sentences to help to improve understanding and recall
- break tasks down into smaller steps (Ambalu, 1977)
- use creative media such as drawing, painting, modelling and music to elicit feelings and emotions
- use life story work (Hewitt, 2000; Hussain, 1997)
- use drama (Shirtliffe, 1995)
- use language that is simple and concrete and vary the way(s) in which information is given
- use audio tape information so that individuals can take it away with them.

Such approaches will enable the professional to involve the individual as much as possible (and as much as they wish) in their own care and any subsequent treatment.

As with bereavement, people with learning disability experiencing a palliative illness are often totally disempowered. They are often not told of their illness (or the extent of their illness) and are frequently not actively involved in their treatment, largely because of the challenges this produces and the existence of negative, overprotective attitudes.

Palliative care and death in a carer   People with a learning disability who are faced with the palliative illness (and eventual death) of their primary carer often experience a whole host of additional challenges as they cope with the multiple losses associated with the death (Box 6.2). Sadly such situations are not uncommon, and the death of a primary carer might initiate many losses for people with learning disabilities, as indicated in Figure 6.1.

Such potential losses can be minimised when palliative care is involved since the outcome (death) is often anticipated, and hence can be constructively planned for, and the sudden consequences minimised for the person with a learning disability who is left behind to

Figure 6.1
Multiple losses
associated with death
of a primary carer

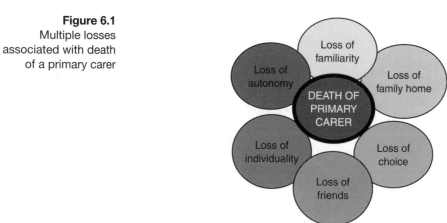

Box 6.2

The death of a carer

Sarah was a disabled woman living at home with her father. His death meant a complete change of lifestyle, as she had to pack a suitcase within an hour of his admission (and subsequent death) to hospital and move into a large unit for people with learning disabilities some 10 miles from her home town.

She never returned to the family home and simultaneously left the day centre that she had attended for many years. For Sarah, the loss of her father brought other multiple losses, all of which needed to be coped with at the same time.

---

cope. This involves agencies such as health and social services and the private sector working together in a proactive way before the inevitable death occurs.

A whole spectrum of professionals and agencies can be involved in palliative care provision and support of the person with a learning disability, including the GP, district nurses, Macmillan nurses, hospice day care, ethics committee (for example in informed consent issues or for those withdrawing from active treatment), dieticians, counsellors, advocates, chaplains, hospital consultants and specialists, solicitors and funeral directors. This is an incredible number to cope with, particularly when the input of individual professionals might increase or decrease over time. For the person who lives in a community home being cared for by professional carers, the central figures to coordinate this care will be the nurses involved. Hence, professional carers need to know who and what services are available and accessible within their local catchment area to support them in caring for the individual who has a palliative care need. They often need to access such specialist help quickly, so preparing for such an event before it is needed would be useful for learning disability nurses.

Needs in palliative care The needs of the individual who has a learning disability and requires palliative care may be similar to those of others who have a palliative illness. Such needs might include:

- a good quality of life until death
- holistic care
- effective pain and symptom management
- to participate in living until dying
- to be treated openly and honestly and with adult status
- counselling and support
- to be cared for by people who can effectively communicate with them
- to be told the truth
- to be cared for by professionals who understand their illness
- to be cared for by professionals who can respond to their needs
- to die in a place of their choosing
- to die with dignity.

In addition to attending to the direct needs of the individual with the palliative illness, care and consideration of, and preparation of, other clients and friends who live in the home alongside the ill person will be important, as will support of any relatives who may wish to be actively involved with the care as the illness progresses. As the illness progresses and becomes more debilitating, the needs of these friends might include:

- acknowledgement of the illness and its potential impact
- an invitation to be actively involved in what is happening around them
- psychological and emotional support
- knowledge and education (what is likely to happen)
- to be treated with honesty, openness and respect
- an opportunity to say their 'goodbyes' to their friend who is ill.

The family need:

- emotional support
- to be kept well informed
- honesty and openness
- an invitation to be actively involved with the care of their loved one.

Again, learning disability nurses should have a pivotal role in acknowledging such needs and in coordinating support systems for others and for themselves. When supporting an individual who requires palliative care, learning disability nurses themselves may need:

- practical help, knowledge and advice
- psychological and emotional support
- educational opportunities
- specialist training.

Supporting an individual through a palliative illness to impending death is no easy task, and collaborative working is the key to effective, meaningful support from an interagency perspective. Learning disability nurses need to learn about palliative care and specialists in palliative care need to learn about learning disability. The learning disability nurse will be the primary coordinator of such care and support services. As when supporting a bereaved individual, there are many challenges that face professional carers as they endeavour to support the individual facing a palliative illness; addressing these challenges will help to untangle the web of uncertainty and help learning disability nurses to be effective, efficient, confident and sensitive carers at such difficult times.

RESPONDING TO THE CHALLENGES

The learning disability nurse may have many roles when supporting the individual with a learning disability in a death, dying or bereavement situation (Read, 1997). Such roles might incorporate:

- **educator**: as professionals help individuals to learn and understand about loss, death and dying
- **active listener**: being available to listen, using the whole body to listen and communicate and not simply the ears
- **communicator**: using alternative communication media such as photographs, picture books and artwork
- **mediator**: talking with parents, relatives and other professionals to enable a consistent approach
- **supporter**: providing active, meaningful support when required
- **advocate**: representing the individual in their needs and their choice to participate in death and dying situations
- **facilitator**: offering options and enabling choice and active participation.

The key role in supporting the bereaved individual who has a learning disability can best be described as one of facilitation (Read, 1999a). This role is very much about involving and enabling the person to participate and engage actively with the process of grief within a positive and supportive environment. The learning disability nurse must utilise a whole range of practical, observational, managerial, communication and interpersonal skills in an effort to involve the individual as much as they wish, and as much as they are able, to participate in the death and dying situation. The key elements of the facilitator role are identified in Box 6.3 (Read, 1999a).

The information in Box 6.3 is offered to guide professional practice towards a consistency of approach when working with bereaved people who have a learning disability. Such an approach serves to address

| Box 6.3 | **Elements inherent in a carer's role: 'facilitation'** |

Finding out what the client knows or needs and identifying what can be done to help; such assessment is crucial to the future support of the client
Acknowledging the loss and its importance and significance to the individual
Communicating simply, clearly and truthfully
Involving the individual as much as possible, and as much as they want to, with what is happening before, during and after death (the opportunity to participate in the rituals surrounding death is very important)
Letting your genuine concern and caring show
Initiating and maintaining respect for the client's need for confidentiality and privacy
Trying alternative methods of communication to help individuals to make sense of what is happening around them—maybe using story books (Hollins and Sireling, 1991a,b) artwork or photographs (Jackson and Jackson, 1999)
Actively listening to the individual, looking for common responses to loss and any perceived difficulty in grieving
Teaching an emotional vocabulary—encouraging the person to use words, draw pictures or paint (for example) to express feelings and emotions
Initiating openness, honesty and sincerity
Offering the individual time; to be there when they need you most
Not forgetting the needs of the family of the person with a learning disability, because they are grieving too.

(Adapted from Read (1999a) by kind permission of Emap Healthcare Ltd.)

and minimise the long-term disenfranchising effects described by Doka (1989), and it may reduce the need for specialist intervention. An important precursor to this facilitating role is the full acceptance that people with learning disability are often exposed to loss and bereavement and do respond to such losses. Such a positive attitude can only serve to enhance and promote the response of professionals to the inherent challenges of the loss and bereavement needs of this client group.

The four-task model (Box 6.4) offered by Fox (1988) is a useful framework when facilitating a healthy grief response. These four tasks

| Box 6.4 | **The four-task model of Fox (1988)** |

Understanding. Information needs to be given according to the ability and needs of the individual and should be in a concrete form where possible (for example using books or pictures; arranging visits).
Expression of feelings. Professional carers should be supportive and encouraging of grieving individuals to nurture self-expression.
Commemoration. There is tremendous value in acknowledging that every life is special and 'sacred'. This uniqueness can be translated into concrete activities or examples (such as photographs or memory books).
Continuation of life. Bereaved people with learning disability need reassurance that it is alright to show a range of feelings, which may not be always extremes of emotion (for example very sad or very happy), and to remember happy times as well as sad times.

can be summed up as acknowledging, responding, supporting and remembering, and they match well with the facilitator role and framework offered in Box 6.3. However, some people with learning disabilities may require additional, more focussed bereavement counselling and support.

THE NEED FOR BEREAVEMENT COUNSELLING AND SUPPORT

The majority of bereaved individuals in society generally find the support they require, at the time they require it, from their own social network, and only a small percentage actually feel the need for specific help from counsellors, psychotherapists or other specialist agencies. Bereaved individuals with a learning disability may find all they require to work through the pain of their loss if they are:

- actively encouraged to participate in the rituals surrounding the death
- encouraged to remember the deceased in a tangible, appropriate way
- offered appropriate, accurate knowledge in a meaningful way
- treated in an open and honest, adult way
- sensitively offered time, space and support to grieve for their loved ones in the way they need.

The key is effective facilitation. However, for some individuals with a learning disability, focussed counselling and support may be required to help them with their grief work. Increasingly, bereavement counselling is being perceived as an alternative to medication or behaviour therapy in support of the bereavement needs of the person with a learning disability. Not every bereaved individual will require such specific therapeutic intervention and Elliot (1995) suggests the following as indicators of specific bereavement counselling needs within this client group:

- those whose anger is high
- those who are profoundly missing the deceased
- those whose social networks are very limited
- those assessed as not coping with their bereavement.

Other indicative factors include the nature or circumstances surrounding the death, the relationship to the deceased, when the death occurred (recently or many years ago), whether the person was allowed to attend the funeral, previous loss experiences and whether the individual is experiencing multiple losses either as a result of, or in addition to, the bereavement.

When the death occurred may be an important issue since some people with learning disabilities may take a long time to accept the finality of the death. Carers need to remain mindful that ambivalence does not necessarily mean that the person does not care and will not miss the deceased person. Full acceptance of the finality of the loss may take some considerable time. It is not uncommon for people with learning disabilities to express sadness and other feelings and responses suddenly 5 or 6 years after the death has occurred. This delayed response may pose problems for several reasons:

1. There has been no record kept of the death.
2. There has been no record kept of the location of the remains of the deceased.
3. There has been no record kept about whether the individual has been told of the death, whether they attended the funeral and what their responses over time have been.
4. Frequent staff movement means that no one remembers that the individual has experienced a bereavement (regardless of the time since the death).

Such a lack of factual and practical information may affect the carer's ability and wish to support the bereaved individual at the time they require it most. Sadly, that wish cannot always be fulfilled (Box 6.5).

Box 6.5	Loss of a history: the story of Mary

Mary was an elderly lady dying of lung cancer. Her dying wish was to be buried with her mother.

No one among the professionals involved in her care was able to discover where her mother had been buried some 70+ years previously. Mary herself had no other living relatives and had no idea when her mother died or where she had lived.

The bereavement guidelines developed by Nottingham Healthcare NHS Trust (2000) address useful ways of recording and storing pertinent bereavement information in a consistent way that enables easy access for professional carers.

Counselling in learning disability

If a person with a learning disability is referred for bereavement counselling, the counsellor would not work in isolation with the client and would recognise the need to involve the professional carer in the overall support strategy of the individual. When the counsellor withdraws (either on a weekly basis or ultimately at the end of the counselling), someone has to be able to continue to support the individual and give them time and space to continue to remember their loved ones in a concrete and positive way. In many cases, this will be the professional carer, and much of the bereavement counsellor's work with the carer will involve:

- offering guidance and knowledge
- giving reassurance and affirmation
- offering ongoing support (where appropriate)
- sharing expertise
- helping carers to manage change effectively
- helping to increase the carer's confidence in dealing with loss and death.

Such support to the carer should not, in any way, affect the confidential relationship between the counsellor and the client, and all bereavement counselling organisations hold explicit guidelines regarding maintaining confidentiality to clarify such potential situations. Accessing a specialist bereavement counselling service may be difficult, as many voluntary counselling agencies are not prepared (either practically or philosophically) to receive people with learning disabilities. However, professionals are beginning to respond to the bereavement needs of this group, resulting in the development of a limited number of services across the UK. The problems of establishing and developing such a specialist bereavement counselling service, from both an organisational and a counselling perspective (including associated data relating to the nature of the clients accessing such a service), are described by Read (2001). Many bereavement counselling organisations use a particular framework or model to guide their counselling practice and to facilitate healthy grief work. Worden's task model (1991), as outlined in Table 6.2, has been a useful framework when supporting the bereaved individual who has a learning disability (Elliot, 1995). The bereavement counsellor's response to Jean (Box 6.1) using Worden's task model is presented in Box 6.6. The bereavement counsellor offered Jean a quiet, confidential and regular space to work through issues

Box 6.6	**Bereavement counselling: the response to Jean's story**

Box 6.1 describes the delayed reaction of Jean to her sister's death. The bereavement counsellor worked with Jean over a period of months, using Worden's (1991) four tasks of grieving as a guide to effective grief work. The list below is a simplified overview of the tasks and approaches used by the bereavement counsellor. It does not identify the specific skills used by the counsellor.

Task one: accept the reality of the loss. This involved finding out about Jean's family, finding out what Jean knew about the death, finding out where the sister was buried, preparing Jean to visit the graveside and eventually taking Jean (with her key worker) to visit the grave and take photographs. Jean decided to construct a memory book of her sister.

> **Task two: work through the pain of grief**. This involved actively encouraging Jean to express emotions and feelings about the death: what she missed most about her sister and how she felt currently; it also involved affirming these responses. Artwork and guided paper exercises were used, including writing a letter to her dead sister to put in the memory book. The counsellor listened to her grief, anger, guilt and sadness.
>
> **Task three: adjust to life without the deceased**. This involved helping Jean to assess her current life, her strengths, her needs and aspirations, her current support system and its effectiveness, and her goals for the future.
>
> **Task four: re-invest in new life**. This involved reviewing the counselling work, affirming achievements, acknowledging future aims and ambitions and planning a healthy and appropriate ending with the counsellor.

associated with her loss. This involved constructing an environment favourable for the development of a relationship between the counsellor and Jean, a crucial element within a cathartic process, and the use of varied approaches. The bereavement counselling involved several key features, including the construction of a life story approach to the bereavement experience, locating the grave, using photographs to relive the burial scene and to prepare for the visit to the grave and accompanying the client to the grave where she placed flowers.

Over a period of months Jean was encouraged to talk about her feelings of loss and sadness, and about her anger at not being allowed to attend the funeral. Jean was given permission to talk about key topics such as her worry about her own death and even to talk to her key worker about planning her own funeral.

A creative response

A bereaved person who also has a learning disability may have distinct specialist needs that are significantly different from those of other non-disabled bereaved people, and carers and bereavement counsellors alike must try to address these needs. This may involve creative approaches and the use of a variety of techniques to promote active engagement, to maximise reciprocal communication and enhance comprehension. This occurs in many contexts but particularly in a loss, death or dying situation.

According to Prout and Stromer (1994, p 7), 'the less articulate client with [sic] mental retardation may feel uncomfortable in verbally orientated sessions'. Consequently, the carer may need to use more concrete methods when offering support from a loss and bereavement perspective. Prout and Stromer (1994) suggest two ways to adapt techniques when working with this client group: to alter the techniques that would be used with clients of the same age but without a learning disability or to use counselling techniques developed for children and adolescents but delivering them in an age-appropriate, socially acceptable way.

For people with learning disability, the bereavement work would initially centre on participating in (and being involved with) the rituals surrounding the death. Afterwards, a huge part of the bereavement work may involve identifying tangible mementos and helping the individual to capture memories of the deceased (see Box 6.4). Methods that may be useful when working with the bereaved individual who has communication and cognition challenges include artwork, life story work, memory books/boxes, pictorial work (books, videos and photographs), drama and poetry, object- and concept-related cue cards and reminiscence work.

Artwork 'The use of colour, paint and design can aid self expression and tension release' (Read, 1999b). There are a number of methods that can help the individual to focus upon something concrete while the carer is encouraging feelings and inner thoughts. These include using family trees, guided exercise sheets to explore feelings and using a blank sheet of paper, paint and colour. The interpretation of any drawing or painting is not seen as being the most crucial outcome; what is important is that it is a safe medium from which to discharge feelings and emotions safely and uniquely.

Life story work Life story work has been used specifically to address bereavement issues with people with learning disabilities (Hussain, 1997) but it also has more generic uses. The important characteristics for effective life story work include client involvement, compiling the work, support in doing the work, ownership (how does the individual know that it belongs to them) and privacy and confidentiality (who has access to the work). Hewitt (2000) explored the effective use of life story approaches for individuals with profound learning disabilities moving from institution to community-based care. Carers used these life books for three purposes: to get to know the person, to define the person and to display the personality of the person. She concludes '... life story work takes the focus away from viewing them as "subjects" or "clients" and considers them as people with their own unique life'. A further advantage to life story work is that it creates a heritage for individuals who often have no recorded histories. The importance of history in the lives of people with learning disability has recently become well documented (Atkinson et al., 1997); from a bereavement perspective, such life stories become invaluable documents.

Memory books/boxes Memory books/boxes are similar to life story books except the focus is very much around a particular memory—often the deceased person. They are a very concrete way of capturing tangible memories and information about the dead person in a very simple, accessible and meaningful way.

Pictorial work Pictorial books, videos and photographs enable clients to engage with complex issues in simple, easy to understand ways. Books such as *When mum died* and *When dad died* (Hollins and Sireling, 1991a,b) can be used proactively (in preparation for an imminent death) or reactively (to explore the individual's bereavement story after the death).

The Speakup video *Coping with death* (Speakup Self Advocacy, 1997) is an excellent resource; it is short, narrated by people with learning disability, simplistically yet powerfully portrayed and often repeats issues to enable comprehension. Again this video can be used proactively, reactively or during group work opportunities and shared learning with people with learning disability.

Photographs are an extremely powerful medium. Jackson and Jackson (1999, p 15) offer short guidelines on effective use of photography from a therapeutic perspective, recommending four broad-based contexts:

- in any client-centred problem-solving exercise
- to reinforce learning, especially when used alongside objects in a teaching programme
- for making choices at any stage and for any level of ability
- to aid reminiscence and to remind.

Photographs can help to make abstract concepts more concrete and real and can be used proactively, reactively or in shared group educational opportunities. Photographs can be easily collected; for example, Figure 6.2 is one of a set of object images used to explain the nature of funerals to an individual with a learning disability: what to expect, what they will see, and identifying symbols such as a coffin, a hearse, the undertakers and an urn. Such photographs provide a simple way to explore understanding (and clarify misunderstanding) of important issues at a difficult time. They can also be used to reconstruct a funeral in pictures, allowing the individual to experience what they had (perhaps) not been allowed to experience or had simply forgotten.

Drama and poetry Drama and poetry can both be used to facilitate emotional expression and explore hidden meanings. Poetry and prose can be extremely powerful and creative ways to capture thoughts and memories of people or places (Read, 1999b).

Object- and concept-related cue cards Object-related (Fig. 6.2) and concept-related (Fig. 6.3) cue cards are fairly simple to construct and can be very powerful and meaningful to people who have limited understanding of difficult concepts.

Figure 6.2
An object-related cue
card. Reproduced by
kind permission of
Sue Read

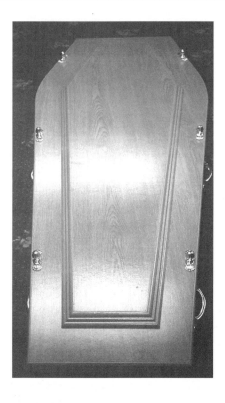

Figure 6.3
A concept-related
cue card. Reproduced
by kind permission of
Jennifer Lauruol

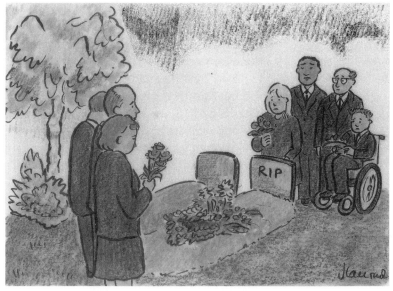

Figure 6.3 is from a set of cue cards designed specifically to explore issues around bereavement and consent to bereavement counselling and research. Again, such cards may be used as a general educative tool, or as an individual aid, either prior to or following a funeral, to

clarify understanding and to explore questions and queries. They can also help the individual to explore feelings and issues associated with their bereavement story.

Reminiscence   Reminiscence work has, according to Stuart (1997, p 9), four functions:

- therapy: coping with change, loss and difficult situations by reflecting on past experience
- advocacy: promoting a cause, understanding processes and feeling confident to challenge systems
- assertiveness: feeling positive about yourself and standing your ground about an issue you have made sense of
- pleasure: sharing experience, valuing your past and participating in enjoyable experiences.

The package by Stuart (1997) is an excellent resource that embraces the concepts of reminiscence and offers practical help in preparing, developing and managing reminiscence generally in the lives of people with learning disability. This package can assist in developing approaches to deal with loss, death and bereavement in those who have learning disabilities. Such approaches have been explored in more detail as part of bereavement counselling by Read (1999b).

EDUCATION, TRAINING AND RECOGNISING THE NEED FOR SUPPORT

Education and training are important from both a client and a carer perspective. Because of the segregated, isolated and institutionalised living experiences of many people with learning disability in the past, many may not have experienced death or participated in the rituals surrounding death. Until leaving the institution, many individuals had never attended a funeral in a hearse but were usually driven to the funeral (often accompanied by several other people with a learning disability) in the hospital minibus. Many individuals never received a condolence card regarding their loved ones. Consequently, Yanok and Beifus (1993) have identified the need for proactive educational opportunities regarding death and dying to prepare individuals specifically for death experiences. This may involve supported educational opportunities, for example visits to cemeteries and undertakers, as part of a long-term planned, educational programme.

Group work appears to be a useful framework within which to address bereavement support specifically (McDaniel, 1989) and loss and change generally (Read et al., 2000), and it can have a very powerful therapeutic impact as individuals share experiences and stories. Sadly, such opportunities are not commonly offered to this client group. However, learning disability nurses can do much to educate and prepare people with learning disability regarding loss, death and bereavement by using deliberate but opportunistic experiences. Carers should take every opportunity to explore feelings, thoughts and responses to human events that occur within the home environment (for example movement of staff or death of pets) and more national events (such as well-known or popular figures who may be seriously ill or who have died and are publicly mourned) in an effort to reinforce the universality of loss, the normality of grief and to nurture and share personal responses.

Professional carers need an understanding of the grieving process. They need knowledge regarding personal responses to loss and complicated grief; they also need an awareness of both individual and social taboos surrounding death so that they can reconcile the difficulties that some carers (including themselves) might have under certain circumstances. Ideally, such carers should have the opportunity to attend multidisciplinary training events where issues surrounding loss, breaking bad news, dying and death can be addressed across professional boundaries, whilst acknowledging and addressing similar personal challenges and responses.

From a palliative care perspective, a percentage of learning disability nurses would benefit from having additional qualifications specifically in palliative care. Both the Diploma and the Degree in Palliative Care are useful qualifications that would enhance the learning disability nurses' existing skills while creating a much-needed specialism in a developing area of work.

Dealing with death and dying is often difficult (Worden, 1991), and the need for managers to recognise this and offer formal ongoing support (and nurture regular, informal ongoing support) is crucial. Written guidelines, philosophy statements of intent and appropriate written recording systems will enable professional carers to develop consistent ways of dealing with death and dying. This should develop alongside support for the professionals involved, such as access to individual clinical supervision, critical debriefing, supervision groups and/or personal counselling.

Not all professional carers will choose to be lead agents within this sensitive topic area, but those who do should be actively supported to develop a sound knowledge base and to develop a wide range of experiences and a range of resources that can be accessed by other professional carers when required. They should also be recognised as having such expertise and have appropriate support and supervision.

FUTURE DEVELOPMENTS

There are a number of impressive developments in the area of loss, death and bereavement (such as the NHS Cancer Screening Programmes

Bereavement (2000) guidelines) but there is room for considerably more creative developments.

More empirical research is needed to identify and clarify the direct needs of the bereaved. Experiences and case studies of individuals experiencing a bereavement make a valuable, human contribution to professional knowledge and understanding and this should continue and be encouraged. Learning disability nurses should be encouraged to write more about the challenges and how they responded in an effort to nurture understanding and clarify practice issues. The development of more literature (for example training packs; therapeutic manuals; cue cards) would support developments and offer consistency of support in practice.

Palliative care Research addressing personal experiences of palliative care and the effectiveness of palliative care interventions would enhance care delivery (Keenan and McIntosh, 2000). More effective methods are needed for assessing pain and managing symptoms, which would improve care management generally. An audit of national palliative care services across geographical regions would offer a baseline indicator of how many palliative services *could* take people with learning disability, how many palliative care services *do* take people with learning disability and what the *uptake* of service actually is. This would assist the development of appropriate and flexible resources to meet the specialist needs of this client group.

Education and training Specialist agencies (such as hospices) need to become more aware of the specialist needs of those with learning disabilities and to prepare their workforce to work collaboratively (and in partnership) with learning disability nurses. Similarly, learning disability nurses need to be better prepared to work in palliative care, and dual qualifications in this area would enhance existing knowledge and skills. Specialist courses need to incorporate and address issues on working with people with communication challenges generally, and learning disability specifically. Collaboration between professionals in different areas could help to ensure that the needs of this group are considered in the planning and development of these courses.

Developing positive practice Good practice and consistency of approach across all disciplines should be encouraged. The checklist in Box 6.7 has been designed for professional carers to assess what services are currently in place from a learning disability, bereavement and palliative care perspective. Specifically, professionals could use it to evaluate current good practice and to identify areas for improvement.

| Box 6.7 | **Developing positive practice in learning disability, bereavement and palliative care** |

The following checklist assesses what services are currently in place.

1. Have any of the staff team attended a course (preferably multidisciplinary) around death, dying or bereavement within the last 2 years? Yes ☐ No ☐

2. Are any of the staff team identified as taking the lead role in loss and bereavement work? Yes ☐ No ☐

3. Do you have easy access to a resource base regarding bereavement support? Yes ☐ No ☐

4. Do you have a client-based recording system where pertinent information can be stored and easily retrieved? Yes ☐ No ☐

5. Do you have easy access to a resource directory regarding how and where to access palliative care information and support for people with learning disabilities? Yes ☐ No ☐

6. Do you have leaflets or other information regarding bereavement or palliative care that you can offer to individuals, families and friends? Yes ☐ No ☐

7. Are any leaflets you have accessible to people with learning disabilities? Yes ☐ No ☐

8. Does anyone in the local palliative care network (for example Macmillan nurses, Marie Curie nurses, hospice, clergy) liaise with the staff team? Yes ☐ No ☐

9. Does anyone in the staff team liaise with the local palliative care network (for example Macmillan nurses, Marie Curie nurses, hospice, clergy)? Yes ☐ No ☐

10. Do you know how to access counselling for people with learning disability in your locality? Yes ☐ No ☐

11. Do you regularly use life story approaches in a client-centred, individual and personal way with people with learning disabilities? Yes ☐ No ☐

12. Does the staff team have easy access to appropriate resources (books, videos, photographs) dealing with loss, bereavement and palliative care? Yes ☐ No ☐

13. Do you have a philosophy statement regarding learning disability, death and bereavement? Yes ☐ No ☐

14. Do you have guidelines regarding bereavement care and support? Yes ☐ No ☐

15. Do you have guidelines regarding palliative care and support? Yes ☐ No ☐

16. Do you have information and contact names and addresses of different cultural, religious and ethnic groups within your locality? Yes ☐ No ☐

17. Do you have an evaluation system in place to monitor this work in a systematic and formal way? Yes ☐ No ☐

CONCLUSIONS This chapter has identified the many issues involved in loss, death and bereavement particularly those impinging on a nurse supporting individuals who have a learning disability. Loss and responses to loss have aspects that are common to all in society and aspects that are specific to those with a learning disability. Working with disability, death and dying is challenging and requires consideration of the needs of many groups: people with learning disabilities, their relatives, their friends and their professional carers. Palliative care is a particular area of need and one in which communication is a key issue. Individuals with a learning disability are affected when palliative care is needed for either themselves or other significant people in their lives.

People with a learning disability will continue to experience the sad business of death and dying, and professionals have to address how best to serve and support them during such experiences. Learning disability nurses will continue to have a pivotal role in coordinating and delivering palliative care; they also have a key role in facilitating healthy grief work to maximise personal growth, develop positive coping strategies and minimise distress.

REFERENCES Ambalu S 1997 Communication. In: O'Hara J, Sperlinger A (eds) Adults with learning disabilities: a practical approach for health professionals. Wiley, Chichester

Atkinson D, Jackson M, Walmsley J 1997 Forgotten lives: exploring the history of learning disability. BILD, Kidderminster

Bimh E, Elliot I 1982 Conceptions of death in mentally retarded persons. Journal of Psychology 3: 205–210

Bonell-Pascual E, Huline-Dickens S, Hollins S et al. 2000 Bereavement and grief in adults with learning disabilities: a follow-up study. British Journal of Psychiatry 175: 348–350

Bowlby J 1996 Attachment and loss: loss, sadness and depression. Basic Books, New York

Bycroft L 1994 Care of a handicapped woman with metastatic breast cancer. British Journal of Nursing 3(3) 126–133

Clarke L, Read S 1998 Bereavement support for people with learning disabilities. Nursing Times 94(28): 51–53

Conboy-Hill S 1992 Grief, loss and people with learning disabilities. In: Waitman A, Conboy-Hill S (eds) Psychotherapy and mental handicap. Sage Publications, London, pp 150–170

Cooley M E 1992 Bereavement care: a role for nurses. Cancer Nursing 15(2): 125–129

Crick L 1988 Facing grief. Nursing Times 84(26): 61–63

Department of Health 1989 Caring for people. HMSO, London

Department of Health 1995 The health of the nation: a strategy for people with learning disabilities. HMSO, London

Doka K 1989 Disenfranchised grief: recognising hidden sorrow. Lexington Books, Toronto, Canada

Elliot D 1995 Helping people with learning disabilities to grieve. Nursing Times 91(43): 209–213

Emerson P 1977 Covert grief reactions in mentally retarded clients. Mental Retardation 15(6): 44–45

Fisher M, Warman J 1990 Bereavement and loss: a skills companion. National Extension College, Cambridge

Fox S 1988 Good grief: helping groups of children when a friend dies. New England Association for the Education of Young Children, Boston, MA

Hewitt H 2000 A life story approach for people with profound learning disabilities. British Journal of Nursing 9(2): 90–95

Hollins S, Sireling L 1991a When dad died. St George's Hospital Medical School, London

Hollins S, Sireling L 1991b When mum died. St George's Hospital Medical School, London

Holmes T, Rahe R 1967 The social re-adjustment rating scale. Journal of Psychomatic Research 11: 213–218

Howells G 1997 A general practice perspective. In: O'Hara J, Sperlinger A (eds) Adults with learning disabilities: a practical approach for health professionals. Wiley, Chichester, pp 61–91

Hussain F 1997 Life story work for people with learning disabilities. British Journal of Learning Disabilities 25: 73–76

Jackson E, Jackson N 1999 Learning disability in focus: the use of photography in the care of people with a learning disability. Jessica Kingsley, London

Keenan P, McIntosh P 2000 Learning disabilities and palliative care. Palliative Care Today 9(1): 11–143

Kerr M, Fraser W, Felce D 1996 Primary health care needs for people with a learning disability. British Journal of Learning Disabilities 24: 2–8

Kitching N 1987 Helping people with mental handicaps cope with bereavement: a case study with discussion. Mental Handicap 15: 60–63

Klass D, Silverman P R, Nickman S L 1996 Continuing bonds: new understandings of grief. Taylor and Francis, Washington, DC

Kloeppel D A, Hollins S 1989 Double handicap: mental retardation and death in the family. Death Studies 13: 31–38

Kubler-Ross E 1969 On death and dying. Macmillan, London

Lindemann E 1944 Symptomatology and management of acute grief. American Journal of Psychiatry 48: 101–141

Lindop E, Read S 2000 District nurses' needs; palliative care for people with learning disability. International Journal of Palliative Nursing 6(3): 117–122

Machin L 1998 Looking at loss: bereavement counselling pack. Pavilion, Brighton

McDaniel B A 1989 A group work experience with mentally retarded adults on the issues of death and dying. Journal of Gerontological Social Work 13(3/4): 187–191

NHS Cancer Screening Programmes 2000 Good practice in breast and cervical screening for women with learning disabilities. NHSCSP Publications, Sheffield

Nightingale J, Ditchfield H, Pepperrel P, Murphy J, Gee P 1998 Meeting the health needs of people with learning disabilities: a comparative study. Mental Health Care 21(21): 60–62

Nottingham Healthcare NHS Trust 2000 Bereavement Guidelines. Highbury Hospital, Nottingham

Oswin M 2000 Am I allowed to cry?, 2nd edn. Souvenir Press, London

Parkes C M 1975 Bereavement: studies of grief in adult life. Penguin, Harmondsworth, UK

Prout H T, Stromer D C 1994 Counselling and psychotherapy with persons with mental retardation and borderline intelligence. Clinical Psychology Publishing Counselling, Vermont

Ray R 1978 The mentally handicapped child's reaction to bereavement. Health Visitor 51: 333–334

Read S 1996 Helping people with learning disabilities to grieve. British Journal of Nursing 5(2): 91–95

Read S 1997 A sense of loss: working with loss and people who have a learning disability. Nursing Standard: RCN Update Learning Unit 071: 11–36

Read S 1998 The palliative care needs of people with learning disabilities. International Journal of Palliative Nursing 4(5): 246–251

Read S 1999a Bereavement and people with a learning disability. Nursing Times Books, Emap Healthcare, London

Read S 1999b Creative ways of working when exploring the bereavement counselling process. In: Blackman N (ed) Living with loss: helping people cope with bereavement and loss. Pavilion, Brighton, pp 9–13

Read S 2001 A year in the life of a bereavement counselling and support service for people with learning disabilities. Journal of Learning Disabilities 5(1): 19–33

Read S, Papakosta-Harvey V, Bower S 2000 Using workshops on loss for adults with learning disabilities. Groupwork 12(2): 6–26

Service K P, Lavoie D, Herlihy J E 1999 Coping with losses, death and grieving. In: Janicki M P, Dalton A J (eds) Dementia, aging, and intellectual disabilities. Taylor and Francis, Washington, DC, pp 330–351

Shirtliffe D 1995 Dramatic effect. Nursing Times 7(23): 62–63

Speakup Self Advocacy 1997 Coping with death. [Video] Speak Up Advocacy, Rotherham

Stroebe M, Schutt H 1996 The dual process model for coping with grief. Keynote paper presented at the third St George's dying, death and bereavement course. St George's Hospital Medical School, London

Stuart M 1997 Looking back, looking forward—reminiscence with people with learning disabilities. Pavilion, Brighton

Tuffrey-Wijne I 1997 Palliative care and learning disabilities. Nursing Times 93(31): 50–51

Weston R, Martin T, Anderson Y (eds) 1998 Loss and bereavement: managing change. Blackwell Science, London

Worden J W 1991 Grief counselling and grief therapy: a handbook for the mental health practitioner, 2nd edn. Tavistock/Routledge, London

World Health Organization 1990 Technical report series 804. World Health Organization, Geneva

Yanok J, Beifus J A 1993 Communicating about loss and mourning: death education for individuals with mental retardation. Mental Retardation 31(3): 144–147

7

Community care: opportunities, challenges and dilemmas

Lesley Styring

OVERVIEW A 'person-centred approach to care', by definition, means having the individual at the heart of the process: taking on board a person's needs but also acknowledging their hopes, dreams and aspirations (Department of Health, 2001). Though ideal, this philosophy is difficult to uphold when the individual concerned has a learning disability, not just because of their intellectual impairment but also because of the associated communication difficulties, which often compound the situation. While it is now good practice to involve people in the decision-making process, some commentators argue quite rightly that much more could be done to engage clients and carers in a meaningful way despite the difficulties that exist (NHS Executive Trent, 2001). This will be a recurring theme throughout this chapter and is discussed in terms of changing practice and the opportunities, challenges and dilemmas practitioners face when working in a community-centred system.

CHANGES IN SERVICES There have been phenomenal changes in learning disability services in recent years, with the closure of large institutions, greater emphasis on social care, increased reliance on primary care and the development of specialist health services (Department of Health, 1997, 1998a,b, 2000a, 2001; Department of Health and Social Security, 1971, 1987; NHS Executive, 1998). There has also been a steady influx of professionals from other disciplines into learning disability services, in growing recognition that the client group has a multiplicity of needs that require specialist input (Thompson and Mathias, 1992). The same case scenario (Box 7.1) is used throughout the text to illustrate different trends in care, to discuss the value of multidisciplinary involvement and to consider the implications of recent government legislation on working practices.

Box 7.1	**Maureen**

Maureen is a woman with moderate learning disabilities and limited communication skills. She presents as someone who is much more capable than she really is; her trusting disposition makes her very vulnerable.

Although Maureen has never married, she gave birth to a daughter in her teens. Contact with her daughter and with other family members is extremely limited.

Maureen has epilepsy in the form of tonic–clonic seizures. These tend to occur in clusters and are thought to be stress related. Maureen was extremely active until approximately 18 months ago when she developed an ulcerated leg. This is obviously causing her a great deal of discomfort and affecting her mobility.

Services at the start of the 20th century

In order to appreciate how far we have progressed in the delivery of services to people with a learning disability, we must consider what life would have been for someone like Maureen had she been born 100 years ago, when care regimens were very different from now.

Although many people with learning disabilities languished in institutions that were originally intended for the criminally insane (North Derbyshire Community Health Care Service (NHS Trust), 1995), there were those who would have been supported and cared for in the community. Rumours about life in the 'asylum' might well have deterred carers from seeking help; for these families there was no possibility of respite care other than that provided by family and friends. People with learning disabilities were excluded from the educational system and there was no alternative daytime provision for them to access. In reality, people like Maureen were often socially isolated and totally reliant on informal carers to meet their needs.

The eugenics movement of the early 1900s advocated sexually segregated institutions to prevent people with learning disabilities procreating and 'lowering' the intelligence of the human race (Hattersley et al., 1987) This, together with society's moral stance on illegitimacy, would have made life very uncomfortable for Maureen. What happened to her and her baby was largely dependent on the reaction of carers, family and the local community where she lived, but many women with learning disabilities were sent to institutions for such 'transgressions'. Maureen would also have been stigmatised because of her epilepsy, which was then attributed to 'demonic' possession (Taylor, 1996) rather than a neurological disorder requiring treatment. The local doctor would have met this and Maureen's other health issues, but again this would have been dependent on the family's financial circumstances and their own health beliefs.

Had Maureen's carers no longer felt in a position to continue the caring role, then the chances are that she would have been compulsorily detained in a large custodial institution under the auspices of the 1913 Mental Deficiency Act. As a person with moderate learning disabilities, Maureen would have probably been categorised as an 'imbecile'. This was defined under the terms of the Act as: 'Persons in whose case there existed from birth or from an early age mental defectiveness not amounting to idiocy, yet so pronounced that they were incapable of managing their affairs or, in the case of children, of being taught to do so' (Ashton and Ward, 1992, p 15). Although the Act was meant to protect and provide asylum for the most vulnerable people in society, it ultimately meant that people with learning disabilities were incarcerated in institutions without any hope of discharge or any formal means of redress.

One can only surmise what it must have been like to live in a large institution, but archive evidence suggests that the principles of the old workhouse regimen still applied. People contributed to the running of the institution by farming and cleaning and regardless of their abilities were 'cared for' rather than rehabilitated. People lived in locked wards and had very little personal space and few possessions. They were made to wear clothes from a communal wardrobe, and 'bundles' of clothes were left ready and waiting for the following morning. Meals were somewhat mediocre: porridge or bread and dripping for breakfast, meat and potatoes for dinner and bread and cheese for tea. People were expected to bathe at certain times; sleep in long dormitories and retire to bed by 7.00 p.m. whether they wanted to or not (North Derbyshire Community Heath Care Service (NHS Trust), 1995). The whole ethos was about care and protection; the reality was that everyone was treated in the same way, irrespective of their individual needs or requirements.

Services in the second half of the 20th century

It was not until the late 1940s, with the development of the welfare state, that institutions were brought under the direction of the National Health Service (NHS). As a consequence, institutions became 'hospitals for the mentally subnormal' and staff who had been attendants in the institution suddenly became nurses, accountable to consultant psychiatrists (Brigden and Todd, 1993). Although these hospitals catered for the patients' physical needs, institutional practices were still rife and specialised treatment was based on general principles pertaining to a specific condition. For example, patients who had epilepsy were taken to another ward and made to sleep on 'epileptic beds' a few inches from the floor, irrespective of the type and frequency of their seizures. Pharmacology was still in its infancy and the choice of anticonvulsant drugs was limited to either phenobarbital or phenytoin. On reflection, it could be argued that coming under the umbrella of the NHS perpetuated the idea that people with learning disabilities were vulnerable and in need of care and attention, rather than promoting their independence and choice.

The move towards a more social model of care actually began with the introduction of the 1959 Mental Health Act, which stipulated conditions under which mentally ill and mentally handicapped people could be detained in hospital. This meant that the majority of individuals previously detained under the terms of the 1913 Mental Deficiency Act now had informal status and could be discharged from hospital. The impact of this Act should not be underestimated, as it paved the way for care in the community. However, it must also be said that patients were unlikely to be aware of their informal status and the fact that they were, in theory at least, free to leave the hospital environment.

At the same time, changes were taking place in Scandinavia that were to have a profound effect on future service developments. The concept of *normalisation* was written into Danish law in 1959, the aim of which was to 'create an existence for the mentally retarded as close to normal living conditions as possible' (Bank-Mikkelsen, 1980). While Denmark and Scandinavia became pioneers in terms of community living, other countries, including Britain, remained relatively unaffected by this new philosophy. Hospitals for the mentally subnormal continued to operate in the UK very much as before; patients were subjected to ritualistic practices, the same daily routines and generalised care strategies.

If we were to reflect on the development of services for people with learning disabilities, we would probably agree that significant events in the 1960s spurred the community care debate. In his book on asylums, Ervine Goffman (1968) discussed the effects of institutionalisation on the individual. He concluded that institutional life had a detrimental effect on the person because daily routines and practices created a dependency on the system. This study, together with a number of disclosures about the scandalous conditions in some mental handicap hospitals, became a catalyst for the closure of long-stay hospitals (Alaszewski and Manthorpe, 1995).

In response to these scandals and the public inquiries that followed (Department of Health and Social Security, 1969), the Government produced a White Paper entitled *Better services for the mentally handicapped* (Department of Health and Social Security, 1971). This proved to be a watershed in service development because it made several major recommendations, including:

- a reduction in the size of the hospital population by means of an active discharge policy
- the development of local social service provision
- greater collaboration between health and local authorities.

To understand the implications of this strategy, the fate of Maureen (Box 7.1) can be considered as an inpatient or as a person living in the community.

Life as a hospital inpatient in the early 1970s

In reality, life for Maureen as an inpatient in hospital in the early 1970s would have been very much the same as earlier in the century. Her life would have revolved around the routines of the day and she would have had very little opportunity to exercise her rights or make choices for herself. Day and recreational activities would have taken place within the hospital grounds, and the former would have probably been something to do with crafts or other similar tasks, with little scope to develop self-help skills. Maureen might have benefited from the refurbishment of the hospital, which was another recommendation from the White Paper (Department of Health and Social Security, 1971), and the development of smaller units away from the large hospital site. For example, heath authorities began developing satellite hostels, primarily for the more able patients as a prelude to them moving out into the community.

However, not everything about institutional life should be discounted or discredited. Indeed one of the positive outcomes of living in a hospital situation was that all the patients received a routine annual medical check up. This was particularly important for people like Maureen who had limited communication skills and were not always able to verbalise how they felt or make their needs known. One must also remember that, at that time, people like Maureen did not have the benefit of speech and language therapists, occupational therapists, physiotherapists or psychologists. The care given was mainly by nursing staff and depended very much on the nurse to identify a person's needs and to follow treatment strategies. While there was a growth in pharmacology and in the choice of sedatives and anticonvulsants that could be used for the client group, some conditions, such as incontinence, mental illness and palliative care, were masked by the learning disability label and not treated.

Life in the community in the early 1970s

If Maureen had not been an inpatient and was living in the community with carers, then there might have been some more noticeable changes in service developments. Local authorities began developing their own provision in terms of hostels and industrial training units, as they were called then. This ultimately meant there was more day care provision for people with learning disabilities living in the community and there were opportunities for respite care. This also marked the beginning of alternative residential care (in the form of group homes). While industrial units can be criticised in terms of the activities that were available, many of the service users valued the opportunity to do what might be considered menial tasks because they considered it to be their 'job'. There was an injustice aspect in doing 'contract work' in terms of exploitation and not being paid adequately for doing a particular task, but this must be balanced against the value many service users derived from being 'employed', and it offered a demarcation between 'work' and recreation.

The Education Act

What was also significant about the early 1970s was the introduction of the Education Act. Children who were previously deemed to be uneducable were brought into the educational system and the onus was placed on local authorities to provide 'special schools' for learning disabled children. As a consequence of this legislation, small schools were built—usually on hospital sites—which were somewhat similar to nursery school provision, with play and music and movement being the main activities provided. Again, with hindsight, it is easy to be critical of such provision. However, at the time, it marked a significant change in attitude because it was no longer considered futile to educate someone with learning disabilities, and it implied that such a person could acquire skills with training and could become much more independent as a result. So, while far from ideal, at least it was a genuine attempt to value children irrespective of their intellectual impairment.

Normalisation

During the 1970s, the moral argument of normalisation began to gain momentum in the USA. Wolfensberger (1972) argued the case for social care and integration in the community on the grounds that the life of a person with learning disabilities should be comparable with that of the 'average citizen'. The principles of normalisation were slow to filter through to some hospitals, but they did lead to attempts to alter the environment by creating flats within existing ward areas. Again, while this was not ideal, there was a growing recognition that something should be done to make the hospital environment more homely. Perhaps the most significant development to occur as a result of Wolfensberger's social policy was some inclusion of patients in the decision-making process, although this was still very much within the confines of institutional life. For example, people were able to make choices about what clothes they wanted to wear and when to go to bed.

The essence of Wolfensberger's philosophical viewpoint was that society would only afford equal rights to people with learning disabilities when they were seen to be leading culturally normal lifestyles in relation to the rest of society (Hyde, 2000). Wolfensberger elaborated on his original proposition and put forward the concept of social role valorisation, which sought to engage people with learning disabilities in socially valued activities. He argued that services should actively support individuals to achieve this aim. In some respects, Wolfensberger fuelled the community care debate further, and the King's Fund (1980) defined three principles for 'ordinary living': people with learning disabilities should have the same human value as anyone else and, therefore, the same human rights; they should have the right to live like others in the community; and they should be treated as individuals by service providers rather than as a homogeneous group.

Another influential commentator was John O'Brien (1987), who devised a list of benchmark accomplishments for learning disability services. Service providers should demonstrate *respect* for people with learning disabilities by:

- creating opportunities for them to engage in meaningful activities that project a positive image
- upholding the right of *community presence*, enabling people with learning disabilities to live in ordinary domestic settings
- upholding the right to have *relationships* with whoever they choose
- promoting *choice* and *personal competence*, which would enable people with learning disabilities to take up and enjoy the services that are provided in the community.

ADDRESSING COMPLEX NEEDS All the philosophies discussed above arose from the debate on community care and served the populace well in terms of closing long-stay institutions and promoting social inclusion. However, it could be argued that the time has come to look beyond these philosophies, and that by treating people with learning disabilities as 'normal' we are in some respects doing them a disservice. Indeed many of them, like Maureen, have complex problems that need to be recognised and, even more importantly, acknowledged and addressed.

During the 1970s and 1980s, there were several government publications that reviewed the progress made since the 1971 White Paper (Department of Health and Social Security, 1978, 1980) and helped to provide a framework for learning disability services (Department of Health and Social Security, 1984; Mental Health Act, 1983). While there had been some attempts to reduce the hospital population and close long-stay hospitals, it seemed that the biggest hindrance to the development of community care was the lack of adequate funding and the division between the NHS and Social Services. In order to overcome this, all the reports recommended greater collaboration between the two main service providers and the use of joint planning and funding to provide more localised service provision.

In retrospect, the recommendations made in the government reports of the 1970s and early 1980s were a prelude to the guidance made in *Caring for people: community care in the next decade and beyond* (Department of Health, 1989a). This White Paper emphasised the fact that the needs of most people with learning disabilities are social rather than health related and, therefore, social services should become the lead agency for purchasing packages of care. It also advocated greater collaboration with the voluntary and independent sector. The White Paper, and the NHS and Community Care Act 1990 that followed, significantly changed the way services for people with learning disabilities were developed and consolidated the shift of emphasis from care in large institutional settings to care in the community (Matthews, 1996a). Alongside this, specialist learning disability services developed to deal with specific problems such as challenging behaviour and dual diagnosis.

A multidisciplinary approach

People with learning disabilities often have a multiplicity of needs that require specialist input (NHS Executive, 1998) and the value of a multidisciplinary approach for this client group cannot be underestimated. Therapy professions came into learning disability services relatively recently. During the 1970s and 1980s, it was mainly the community learning disability nurse and social worker who took the lead in providing support for people with learning disabilities and their carers. However, since the mid-1980s, there has been a steady influx of other professionals into the service (NHS Executive, 1998). Although community learning disability teams vary in composition, they tend to include:

- community learning disability nurses
- consultant psychiatrists
- speech and language therapists
- occupational therapists
- physiotherapists
- psychologists
- social workers.

This means that the person with learning disabilities can benefit from a wide range of expertise and support to enhance their quality of life. A multidisciplinary approach to Maureen's situation (see Box 7.1) would probably need to involve all members of the community learning disability team.

Community learning disability nurse

The community learning disability nurse plays a pivotal role and would work in collaboration with Maureen, her carers, members of the community learning disability team, colleagues in primary care and day centre staff to make sure her needs were properly addressed. A nursing assessment would be undertaken using either a recognised nursing model such as the *Activities of daily living* (Roper et al., 1990) or a health surveillance tool such as *The okay health check* list (Mathews, 1996b); both of these give an indication of health issues requiring further action. In Maureen's case, a nursing assessment would highlight issues relating to her epilepsy, mobility and pain control, but it should also take into account conditions that may have hitherto been overlooked, such as cardiovascular problems and mental illness. Once Maureen's needs had been identified, the community learning disability nurse would be responsible for devising, implementing and evaluating care plans, which in this case would probably focus on Maureen's epilepsy and ulcerated leg.

The role of the community learning disability nurse is very diverse. Promoting health and well-being is core business and, as well as working on an individual basis with clients, the nurse will often facilitate specialist support groups either alone or in collaboration with other colleagues. As well as offering advice on health issues, the community learning disability nurse may be involved in risk management, mental health promotion, parenting support, palliative care and rehabilitation. Counselling is another area of expertise and, for someone like Maureen, the community nurse might help with anxiety management (to improve the epilepsy) and bereavement (in relation to the loss of a child). The community learning disability nurse also has a part to play in developing personal competence; again, for someone like Maureen, this may involve increasing self-help skills and dealing with issues of consent.

Speech and language therapist A speech and language therapist would be able to assess Maureen's communication skills and level of verbal comprehension. This is extremely important to enable individuals with communication problems to make informed choices and be actively involved in decisions about their care. Any deficits in conversational skills, listening skills, auditory skills and understanding could inevitably lead to a breakdown in communication. If Maureen was unable to express herself verbally, then she would be an unequal partner in discussions and it would be hard for her to make choices for herself without a lot of support. A speech and language assessment would enable practitioners to relate to Maureen much better, by knowing how to present information effectively and what format to use.

Psychologist Maureen's limited communication skills and poor level of understanding make her extremely vulnerable and bring into question her ability to give informed consent. This is often an area of considerable concern for practitioners, who are caught between protecting vulnerable people and wanting to preserve their rights. If there is any doubt about a person's ability to give consent, a request can be made for psychometric tests to assess their level of mental impairment (Tulsky et al., 1998; Wechsler, 1991), social skills (Sparrow et al., 1984) and the presence of mental health problems (Derogatis, 1993; Prosser et al., 1993). A psychologist would be able to determine Maureen's level of understanding in terms of the decision-making process, and whether or not she could legally consent to medical treatment or sexual relationships. If Maureen did not have the capacity to make decisions for herself, she would have to be viewed as a vulnerable adult and there would have to be some strategy for managing her medical treatment and to protect her from possible abuse and exploitation.

Consultant psychiatrists Maureen might well attend a specialist outpatient clinic for advice and support regarding her epilepsy. Although it is estimated that 40% of people with learning disabilities have epilepsy, and the incidence increases with the severity of the impairment (Cunningham and Zaagman, 2000), very few of them actually attend specialist clinics at the neurology department. Instead it is often specialist learning disability services and consultant psychiatrists who offer advice and treatment with regards to epilepsy. Advancements in the treatment of epilepsy have been phenomenal in recent years, with more accurate diagnostic techniques and greater choice of drugs. However, while the aim is to control the epilepsy with the least possible amount of drugs, for many people with learning disabilities monotherapy is often difficult to achieve.

Social worker A social worker might well be involved in Maureen's case and as such would be obligated to undertake a full needs assessment in accordance with the recommendations made in the NHS and Community Care Act 1990. The social worker would need to consider whether or not Maureen could access community resources and, if not, whether services could be adapted to meet her needs. Consideration would also need to be given to Maureen's social networks and what support was available from the family to enable her to live as independently as possible in the community. The social worker would be instrumental in co-ordinating activity to make sure that issues identified in the care plan were being addressed. If Maureen was still living at home with carers, the social worker could be involved in organising respite care either for a designated period in a respite care facility or in terms of day care. If Maureen and her family were requesting alternative residential care provision, then the social worker would play a lead role in trying to find suitable accommodation.

Community living options   Community living options for people with learning disabilities vary from area to area and can include provisions on hospital sites, supported living schemes, residential and nursing homes and village communities. Some people with learning disabilities have their own tenancy agreements with housing associations and others are cared for and supported by charitable organisations or independent providers. The last group has had a major impact on service provision in relation to the type of accommodation being provided. Indeed, some very large residential and nursing homes have more than 40 beds, central kitchens and lots of routines, which are akin to an institution. This obviously presents many challenges. How do we prevent people with learning disabilities being put into larger and larger institutions? How do we maintain a quality of service in the independent sector? How do we ensure individual rights are upheld? Other concerns are the variation in quality and cost of residential services (Emerson et al., 1999) and client choice versus best value.

SERVICE AT THE END OF THE 20TH CENTURY   As can be appreciated from the above discussion, services for people with learning disabilities are now hugely different from what they were 100 years ago. Hospitals have contracted and closed and specialist services have been developed in response to the increased number of people with complex medical needs, challenging behaviour and dual diagnosis. Many people with learning disabilities have additional health problems that can go undetected and undiagnosed (Mencap, 1998) and learning disability nurses have been proactive in health surveillance, health education and health promotion. They have also begun to develop a particular interest in specific areas of learning disability, such as epilepsy, palliative care, parenting and the criminal justice system. It is fair to say that a lot of services have developed out of personal interest; the question is whether service plans should become increasingly specialised or whether developments should be allowed to happen in an ad hoc way.

Role of primary care   Developments in specialist learning disability services cannot be viewed in isolation. Rather they must be considered in conjunction with developments in primary care, as these changes have had, and continue to have, a major impact on people with learning disabilities and their carers. The whole ethos behind the NHS reforms following the NHS and Community Care Act 1990 was to generate income that could then be used to provide better quality services. The introduction of GP Fund Holding and the creation of Acute and Community Trusts (Department of Health, 1989b) were meant to improve efficiency and make primary health care more responsive to the needs of the local population. In reality, the internal market resulted in 'unhealthy' competition between NHS service providers, with very little sharing of ideas and good practice. Specialist learning disability services had to respond not only to the needs of social services but also to those of GP fund holders and their colleagues in primary care. Equally, primary health-care teams have had to respond to an increased number of people with learning disabilities living in the community.

Since being elected into office, the Labour administration has introduced further reforms to modernise the NHS. In the initial White Paper *The new NHS: modern dependable* (Department of Health, 1997), the Government stated its intention to replace the internal market with integrated care based on partnership, thus removing some of the rivalries and competition between services. GP Fund Holding was to be replaced by Primary Care Groups, which, in turn, would later become Primary Care Trusts. These self-governing organisations would be charged with maintaining and developing localised health services that meet national and local requirements. The relevance of these changes for people with learning disabilities is that specialist services are now in the process of reconfiguration. Some are aligning themselves with mental health services and forming combined trusts; others are merging with social services and still others are working towards becoming care trusts in their own right. Practitioners are establishing a Primary Care Trust focus and are adapting their working practices in response to changes in primary care.

Health promotion and disease prevention

Other government initiatives in recent years have aimed to improve the health of the populace through health promotion and disease prevention (Department of Health, 1992, 1997, 1998a,b). Although the recommendations made in earlier publications helped to localise resources, the onus was very much on the individual to be responsible for personal health and well-being. There was great variation in NHS provision from area to area, and the underlying causes of ill-health such as poverty, poor housing and unemployment were not readily addressed. In response to growing concerns about public health, the Labour Government introduced several strategies including health improvement programmes and national service frameworks (Department of Health, 2000a). These were designed to tackle inequalities in health and reduce the incidence of certain diseases (Department of Health, 1999) using a concerted multi-agency approach involving health, social services, education, housing and employment agencies. Again, this has particular relevance for people with learning disabilities because of their associated health conditions and the fact that many of these individuals and their carers are at significant risk in terms of living in poverty and being unemployed.

Policy for learning disability

The recent White Paper *Valuing people: a new strategy for learning disability for the 21st century* (Department of Health, 2001) set out the Government's proposals to improve the lives of people with learning disabilities and their carers. The four key principles that underpinned the document were:

- legal and civil rights
- independence
- choice
- inclusion.

The whole ethos of the White Paper was about citizenship and the rights of people with learning disabilities to be valued members of society. People with learning disabilities face discrimination on a daily basis and the White Paper clearly indicated that everything should be done to prevent this and that measures should be taken to uphold their legal and civil rights. Promoting independence and choice were key aims and person-centred planning featured very strongly throughout the document to ensure that people with learning disabilities have some control over their own destiny. The other key theme of the White Paper was social inclusion. People with learning disabilities should be able to access mainstream services rather than remain on the periphery of social integration and community participation.

The White Paper was explicitly linked to other government initiatives aimed at reducing inequalities in health (Department of Health, 1999). The interface between primary and specialist care was also acknowledged, and while the onus was on primary care there was recognition that health facilitators are needed to assist people with learning disabilities to access mainstream services. One of the specific initiatives proposed by the White Paper was the development of *health action plans* for every individual with a learning disability. The health facilitator would have a pivotal role in devising these plans in partnership with the primary care team. The plans would be updated at times of significant life events, for example at times of transition and on leaving home.

Accessing mainstream services

Although much has been made in recent years of the need to develop a seamless service between health and social care, there is a strong case for the main partnership for specialist learning disability services being with primary care. The ability of people with learning disabilities to access mainstream services is obviously important, but unless this is done with the support of specialist services, and community nurses in particular, the health-related needs of people with learning disabilities will continue to be overlooked. Colleagues in mainstream services lack knowledge about the client group, and it would be nonsensical to expect generic services to be able to meet their needs immediately.

Indeed if this were to be the case, there would be a human resource issue in terms of taking staff away from mainstream work to do interventions specific to learning disability. A case in point would be pain assessment. This is obviously a much more lengthy process when the person has learning disabilities, and it can take anything up to 3 hours compared with the average 20 minutes. Everything takes longer; the consultation process is more involved and, in reality, access to mainstream services is harder. The rhetoric of the White Paper is right provided that service providers can back it up.

Accessing specialist services

Another worry is that generic services will become an excuse for not having specialist services and the role of the registered learning disability nurse will once again be brought into question because commissioners and providers think mainstream services can be everything to all people. However, as people with learning disabilities access generic services, their specialist needs will become more apparent and there will be an even greater need to invest in registered learning disability nurses who can focus on more specialist activities, thereby complementing the work of other health professionals. Registered learning disability nurses need to be proactive rather than reactive to change; they should be supported in terms of training and education to allow their role to evolve naturally rather than being based on past requirements.

Employment opportunities

It will be interesting to see how specialist learning disability services develop in response to the Government's clear intent to give learning-disabled people more employment opportunities and to develop the 'Connexions' service for children in transition (Department of Health, 2001). While not wishing to minimise the value of this policy in terms of equality and promoting self-worth, people with learning disabilities often have associated health problems that could prove a risk in the employment environment. That is not to say they are unemployable, but employers will need a lot of support to accommodate people with learning disabilities. Here again, the learning disability nurse could have a valuable role in offering advice on health-related issues, for example dispelling some of the myths surrounding epilepsy and the use of computers so that people with epilepsy can do this type of work.

Supporting parents with learning disabilities

In recent years, there has been a marked increase in the number of parents with a learning disability and this trend looks set to continue. While it is a fundamental right for people with learning disabilities (such as Maureen, Box 7.1) to have children of their own (Human Rights Act 1998), there are many associated issues such as providing appropriate levels of support and multiprofessional involvement. The White Paper argues that parents with learning disabilities should be properly supported and there should be close collaboration between child and adult services, midwives and health visitors (Department of Health, 2000b; English, 2000). Unfortunately for many parents with learning disabilities, child rearing goes into the realms of child protection and risk management. While the safety of the child is always paramount, the White Paper acknowledges that there are deficits in the current system; for example, most parents are assessed by social services and not by a specialist in learning disability. This often leads to children being taken into care. Social workers do not always have sufficient understanding of learning disability and the right approaches to parenting skills; consequently, a specialist role may well develop in supporting people with learning disabilities to ensure that they have the same opportunities as other parents. This will probably mean that, in future, we have specialist nurses who assist midwives, health visitors and other staff such as the child protection team.

Defining who can access learning disability services

Another issue relates to the client group. The White Paper is quite specific about who should be able to access specialist learning disability services and it excludes individuals on the periphery of services who had been seen previously, for example people with mild learning disabilities and mental health problems and those with certain types of autism such as Asperger's syndrome. This is obviously a cause for concern, particularly with the former, who have often been passed from one service to another without having their needs properly addressed. In addition, increasing numbers of children with profound disabilities requiring acute clinical nursing are surviving into adulthood; this again has implications for both specialist and primary care in terms of the skills needed to provide good quality care.

Implementing person-centered planning

To some extent, the success of *Valuing people* (Department of Health, 2001) will largely depend on the tripartite relationship between person-centred planning, advocacy and the uptake of Direct Payments. Implementation of person-centred planning will be one of the biggest challenges for service providers and practitioners. Some practitioners might argue that they already give a person-centred approach to care in that they focus on the needs of the individual. However, there is a fundamental difference between doing what is perceived to be in the best interests of the person and working in partnership to help the individual attain their goals and dreams. If we consider Maureen's situation again, a person-centred approach to care would necessitate working closely with Maureen and significant others to devise a care plan. In Maureen's case, this may include family members, friends and neighbours as well as the practitioners. A person-centred approach to care should acknowledge the uniqueness of the individual and bring together all key people, with the person being central to the process. As such, the network of support will vary from person to person, and in response to changes in their personal circumstances.

Though ideal, a person-centred approach to care is not always easy to achieve because of the tension that exists between upholding the rights of the individual to make choices for themselves and professional accountability. For example, someone like Maureen is extremely vulnerable and it would be ethically and morally very difficult not to intervene if she was considered to be at significant risk. A community nurse who is bound by a code of professional conduct (Nursing and Midwifery Council, 2002) has a duty to care for the individual and could be deemed negligent for not acting in the person's best interests.

Advocacy Another difficulty is when the person has additional communication problems. The challenge for practitioners is to enable the person to make informed choices when they have difficulty understanding and making their wants and desires known. This is even more problematic if the person concerned has profound disabilities and very limited communication skills. Practitioners often find themselves struggling between 'doing what's right' and upholding the rights of the individual. While people with learning disabilities are beginning to develop skills in self-advocacy, there remains a significant number of people who are unable to challenge decisions for themselves. The dilemma for us as practitioners is how we ascertain their wishes without it being mere tokenism. Some services have made a valiant effort to engage people with learning disabilities in service development and care delivery, but there is recognition that much more can be done, particularly in terms of those less articulate individuals. A person-centred approach for more profoundly disabled people has its challenges but it is an achievable goal with the right knowledge, skills, time and resources.

The whole issue of advocacy is worthy of further exploration and those who have been questioned and challenged by confident service users will know how successful and thought provoking this can be— particularly when the service user has been able to argue the case so eloquently in a 'professional arena'. While more should be done to promote self-advocacy, there is also a case to develop citizen advocacy, but speaking with, as opposed to speaking for. One must also remember that consultation with carers is not necessarily the same as dealing with the person direct. Both groups have very distinct needs and desires, and it is important for practitioners to recognise that these views, though both are valid, can be very different. If the wants and desires of the service user are different from the wants and desires of the immediate carers, this can pose difficulties and tensions for practitioners.

Finance: the Direct Payment scheme

Another area of concern is finance. There are always financial constraints, and choices will need to be made between central planning, which could lead to an inflexible service, and person-centred service, which is personal but costly. The Direct Payment scheme was implemented to allow a person-centred use of funding. There is always going to be potential conflict between what people want and what services can afford. For example, how does a care manager respond to the wishes of a service user who wants to live in a different environment when there is finite budget and limited options? The worry is that person-centred planning becomes elitist and is only truly implemented for a small number of people. The more individualised the care becomes, the more expensive the care package; for those people with very high support needs (as with challenging behaviour) managing their care individually could become horrendously expensive. This also means that there will not be a team of people who can manage complex needs and every problem will be a new problem rather than being 'routine' and 'manageable'.

There is also the question of flexibility. The paradox is that person-centred planning could result in a much more rigid, inflexible service for some people unless service providers combine resources and develop much larger services in order to generate more flexibility in the system. A case in point is Direct Payments. The ability to buy the desired services is highly commendable, but where is the flexibility in the system to cover annual leave, sickness and emergencies? For example, what happens if the worker who is supposedly coming at 7.30 a.m. telephones at 7.00 a.m. to say he cannot come in? This leaves the service user very vulnerable, particularly where their needs fall outside usual working hours. Yet this is exactly what Direct Payments should be for—to give people support when they need it. Help is usually needed in the early mornings, in the evenings and at weekends and these are precisely the times when it is difficult to get cover. A day centre may not be ideal but it is always available to give support. Consequently, it is clear that the Direct Payment system needs to be managed within a network that is large enough to provide emergency cover.

Anecdotal evidence suggests that people with learning disabilities find accessing Direct Payments a lengthy and complicated process; in fact, there is a poor uptake compared with other eligible groups. There is also the added complication of employment law, because the users themselves (albeit with support) are employing people to undertake duties on their behalf. Despite the difficulties that exist, Direct Payments are a means of providing a more person-centred approach and it will be interesting to see how people with learning disabilities make use of and benefit from this initiative in years to come.

CONCLUSIONS When we reflect upon the last 100 years, it is quite apparent that there have been huge changes in learning disability services. While there are still some commonalities, there are to all intents and purposes massive differences in care regimens. In years gone by, the person in our case study, Maureen, would probably have lived in a very large institution with very little community integration and no specialist input. Knowledge and treatment of conditions such as epilepsy was very limited and the person with learning disabilities was a 'passive recipient' of care. Learning disability services have been transformed since the 1970s, with hospital closures, greater emphasis on primary care and the development of specialist health services. The impact of *normalisation* in the 1970s cannot be underestimated, but perhaps the time has come to acknowledge the detrimental effect its continued use may have on people with learning disabilities. To be truly person centred, we must acknowledge the uniqueness of the individual and in doing so acknowledge the fact that they often have very complex needs and additional health issues that need to be addressed. The situation today is hopefully very different. Maureen should have the benefit of a multidisciplinary approach to care and a wide range of community living options to meet her needs. It will be interesting to see what impact *Valuing people* (Department of Health, 2001) will have in years to come. Certainly no one can argue with the philosophical basis on which it was developed. However, there are underlying assumptions that service providers will make good use of person-centred planning, that people with learning disabilities will want Direct Payments and that advocacy services will be available to support them. Yet all three components have been problematic in the past. It will be interesting to see how practitioners and service providers respond to the opportunities and challenges that lie ahead.

There has been a lot of emphasis on partnership in recent years, but for the author the greatest partnership is with learning-disabled people themselves. All of us have hopes, dreams and aspirations, no matter how small or how large they may be, and the challenge for practitioners and service providers in the future is to help people with learning disabilities realise theirs. Person-centred planning should be an integral part of everyday practice. It should not be automatically assumed that it is about helping people with learning disabilities plan for major life events such as moving home. Rather it is about helping them to get day-to-day things that will make life more pleasurable, such as supporting someone to take up a hobby or renew an acquaintanceship. Although intellectual impairments and communication difficulties can make the process harder, improvements can be achieved with proper resources, some creativity and collaborative working.

The Government strategy for people with learning disabilities (Department of Health, 2001) has a lot to commend it and it has the potential to take learning disability services to another dimension. While it should help overcome social exclusion and promote citizenship, practitioners and those charged with implementing the strategy have a lot of barriers to overcome if the changes outlined in the White Paper are to enhance and improve the care of people with learning disabilities. Maureen and others like her should have a very different lifestyle from here on, but the success or failure of the White Paper will only be determined with the passage of time.

REFERENCES

Alaszewski A, Manthorpe J 1995 Goffman, the individual, institutions and stigmatisation. Nursing Times 91(37): 38–39

Ashton G, Ward A 1992 Mental handicap and the law. Sweet and Maxwell, London

Bank-Mikkelson N 1980 Denmark. In: Flynn R J, Nitsch K E (eds) Normalisation, social integration and community services. Baltimore University Park Press, Baltimore, MD, pp 51–70

Brigden P, Todd M (eds) 1993 Concepts in community care for people with a learning difficulty. Macmillan, London

Cunningham O, Zaagman P 2000 Person centred planning. Learning Disability Practice 3(3): 16–19

Department of Health 1989a Caring for people: community care in the next decade and beyond. HMSO, London

Department of Health 1989b Working for patients: the Health Service caring for the 1990s. A summary of the White Paper on the Government's proposals following its review of the NHS. HMSO, London

Department of Health 1992 The health of the nation. HMSO, London

Department of Health 1997 The new NHS: modern, dependable. HMSO, London

Department of Health 1998a A first class service: quality in the new NHS. HMSO, London

Department of Health 1998b Modernising social services: promoting independence, improving protection, raising standards. HMSO, London

Department of Health 1999 Saving lives: our healthier nation. HMSO, London

Department of Health 2000a The NHS plan. The Stationery Office, London

Department of Health 2000b A jigsaw of services. The Stationery Office, London

Department of Health 2001 Valuing people: a new strategy for learning disability for the 21st century (Cm 5086). The Stationery Office, London

Department of Health and Social Security 1969 Report of the Committee of Inquiry into Allegations of Ill-treatment of Patients and Other Irregularities at Ely Hospital, Cardiff (Cmnd 3975). HMSO, London

Department of Health and Social Security 1971 Better services for the mentally handicapped. HMSO, London

Department of Health and Social Security 1978 Helping mentally handicapped people in hospital: a report to the Secretary of State for Social Services by the National Development Group for the Mentally Handicapped. HMSO, London

Department of Health and Social Security 1980 Mental handicap: progress, problems and priorities. HMSO, London

Department of Health and Social Security 1984 Helping mentally handicapped people with special problems: report of a DHSS Study Team. HMSO, London

Department of Health and Social Security 1987 Promoting better health. HMSO, London

Derogatis L R 1993 SCL-90-R symptom checklist-90-R USA. National Computer Systems, Washington, DC

Emerson E, Robertson J, Gregory N et al. 1999 Quality and costs of residential supports for people with learning disabilities summary and implications. Hester Adrian Research Centre, Manchester

English S 2000 Parents in partnership. Learning Disability Practice 3(2): 14–18

Goffman E 1968 Asylums: essays on the social situation of mental patients and other inmates. Harmondsworth, Penguin

Hattersley J, Hosking G P, Morrow D, Myers M 1987 People with mental handicap: perspectives on intellectual disability. Faber and Faber, London

Human Rights Act 1998 HMSO, London

Hyde E 2000 Welfare states. Learning Disability Practice 2(2): 12–16

King's Fund 1980 An ordinary life. King's Fund, London

Mathews D R 1996a Learning disabilities: the challenge for nursing. Nursing Times 92(27): 36–38

Mathews, D R 1996b The Okay Health Check. Fairfield Publications, UK

Mencap 1998 The NHS—health for all? Mencap, London

Mental Deficiency Act 1913 HMSO, London

Mental Health Act 1959 HMSO, London

Mental Health Act 1983 HMSO, London

NHS and Community Care Act 1990 HMSO, London

NHS Executive 1998 Signposts for success. Department of Health, Wetherby

NHS Executive Trent 2001 Learning disabilities in the new NHS: what must we do to improve the profile of services for people with learning disabilities. NHS Executive, Sheffield

North Derbyshire Community Health Care Service (NHS Trust) 1995 The guilded cage—the history of Whittington Hall Hospital 1912–1996. [Video] Active Image, Sheffield

Nursing and Midwifery Council 2002 Code of professional conduct for the nurse, midwife and health visitor. NMC, London

O'Brien J 1987 A guide to lifestyle planning. In: Wilcox B, Bellamy T (eds) A comprehensive guide to the activities catalogue. Paul Brookes, Baltimore, MD

Prosser H, Moss S, Costello H, Simpson N, Patel P 1993 The MiniPAS-Add: an assessment schedule for the detection of mental health problems in adults with developmental disabilities. Hester Adrian Research Centre, Manchester

Roper N, Logan W W, Tierney A J 1990 Using a model for nursing, 5th edn. Churchill Livingstone, Edinburgh

Sparrow S S, Balla D A, Cicchetti D V 1984 Vineland Adaptive Behavior Scales. American Guidance Service, Washington, DC

Taylor M 1996 Managing epilepsy in primary care. Blackwell Science, Oxford

Thompson T, Mathias P 1992 Standards and mental handicap—keys to competence. Baillière Tindall, London

Tulsky D, Zhu J, Ledbetter M 1998 Wechsler adult intelligence scale, 3rd edn. The Psychological Corporation/Harcourt Brace, San Antonio, TX

Wechsler D 1991 Wechsler intelligence scale for children, 3rd edn. The Psychological Corporation/Harcourt Brace, San Antonio, TX

Wolfensberger W 1972 The principle of normalisation in human services. National Institute of Mental Retardation, Toronto, Canada

8 Professional education: foundation for the future

Anne Markwick and Alan Parrish

OVERVIEW
'People with a learning disability are among the most socially excluded and vulnerable groups in the UK today.' These are the opening words in *Valuing people: a new strategy for learning disability for the 21st century* (Department of Health, 2001). This important document sets out the current Government's commitment to improving the lives of people with learning disabilities. It shows how they will meet this commitment by working closely with local councils, health services, voluntary organisations, education providers, housing departments and employment agencies to provide new opportunities for people with a learning disability to lead full and active lives. More importantly, people with learning disabilities and their families will be central and integral in the decision-making process.

This chapter highlights the role that nurses will play in these new and evolving services, and the educational updating needed if they are to be effective, efficient and valued members of the multidisciplinary team. Emphasis is given to the multidisciplinary aspect of the care provided and the consequent need to provide educational opportunities to meet the ongoing needs of staff. While it is obvious that each professional group has particular learning requirements, the essence of good educational programmes has to be the establishing of experiences that cross the boundaries of the professions. The particular responsibilities and accountability of the nurse to the Nursing and Midwifery Council (NMC) are referred to and also the need to pay heed to the requirements of Post Registration Education for Practice (PREP).

The educationalist has a pivotal role in change management and promoting the ethos within *Valuing people* (Department of Health, 2001). Cognisance is given to the Learning Disability Awards Framework and its value in providing a recognised route to qualification and career progression for care workers in learning disability services.

PRE NURSING EDUCATION

A more complex health-care delivery system that is integrated, needs-led and involves users in its planning generates many new challenges. To meet these successfully, it is essential that the preparation and continuing education of staff is paramount. The move from an institutional service to one that is community-based primary care has allowed a more individualised and user-focussed service to be provided for people with a learning disability (Birchenall and Parrish, 1997). Consequently, this group should have, and expect to have, access to the same quality of service as others in the community. The nurse, whether working as part of a community team or in a residential service, has been central to the support and care offered by general practitioners (GPs).

These changes have challenged both nurses and educators in many ways, and innovative further education and training packages are required for a diverse and multiskilled workforce. Major changes have taken place in education provision as nursing has become established on the university campus, and an all-graduate profession is seen as a long-term outcome. These changes have meant that nurses are becoming more highly qualified. There are a wide range of degrees available, relevant to the needs of particular client groups. Courses have become more flexible, and opportunities to select individual modules have made the journey towards a degree both varied and exciting.

Distance learning packages are more available and nurses are adjusting to this new style and type of learning, which enables flexibility in personalised study to be a valued option. For the first time, in 2002, pre-registration nurse education is available through the Open University. There has also been an increase in joint and shared learning opportunities to facilitate educational courses where colleagues from different professional backgrounds join together in a learning experience of each others' contribution to care.

Changing needs in education

The dilemma for managers of services has been the range of professionals involved in the service and the diversity of their educational needs. While the emphasis in practice and in service provision has been on team-building and integrated working, all the professional groups have resisted the move towards generic training, although there has been some progress in the area of postregistration training, where modules of shared learning have been developed. The gap between education and practice has long been debated, with the literature full of suggested solutions, including collaboration, mentorship, preceptorship and joint appointments (Parrish, 2002; UKCC, 1993).

The educational needs of all the professionals changed as the service developed from the custodial and institutional model to encouraging a more ordinary style of living. It is here where nurses and nursing have had the greatest challenge. The traditional lecturer/tutor model, although still preferred in some places, has almost disappeared as the need to demonstrate practice competence has become the established norm. Forward-thinking nurse educators are spending much of their time in the practice areas and influencing standards across the services. This, in turn, challenges and breaks down the theory–practice gap that would be perpetuated if education and service continued to be seen as separate. The development of nurse practitioner roles has also influenced this change. In some areas, these roles are being developed further so that senior level posts such as Director of Nursing are being linked to education posts either in curriculum design and delivery or in research. This can challenge some of the fundamental assumptions often held in education about competence currency within an environment of rapid and radical change. Being both a senior manager within a Trust and a senior educationalist gives a real opportunity to challenge the theory–practice divide and to forge a path of convergence.

Learning disability nursing The primary focus over many years of nurse education in learning disability had been to provide services in a health setting. The range of roles of the professionals in learning disability care, together with the constant changes and developments in service provision, make it essential to plan educational experiences of a multidisciplinary nature to ensure an effective and an efficient use of resources, both financial and workforce. The introduction of Project 2000 and the Diploma level nurse curriculum, which embrace a degree of shared learning before students move to their chosen branches of the profession, has made a good start in preparing nurses to work in a multidisciplinary service. The contribution of some nurses to the development of educational opportunities for unqualified colleagues and informal carers through the Vocational Qualification arena has also enhanced competence. Joint courses are now more common, with a joint nursing and social work degree one of the first examples.

Specialist modules on all aspects of vocational qualifications were developed in large numbers during the 1990s and this has enhanced both competence and confidence in the workforce. *Valuing people* (Department of Health, 2001) had as one of its objectives the introduction of targets for the training of the learning disability workforce: 'From 2002 all new recruits to learning disability care services are to be registered with the Learning Disability Awards Framework (LDAF)…By 2005, 50% of front line staff to have achieved NVQ Level 2'.

The learning disability nurse has led and directed much of the work in setting standards and in quality control across the service, as well as assuming the responsibility in many services for the development of staff within that service.

POST REGISTRATION EDUCATION The benefits of postregistration education are threefold (Pearce, 2001). It helps people to:

- remain professionally accountable
- link to their own personal development plan
- connect to their employer's strategy.

It is almost a triangle. Pearce (2001) cited Howard in advising that, ideally, postregistration education should form an integral part of the nurse's individual annual performance review and ongoing supervision. It should, therefore, identify the professional's own and the employer's current needs, and it should also focus on career development aspirations and opportunities that might develop over time. She emphasised that it needed to be part of a 'grand plan'.

For some time, nurses in certain fields failed to move on from the public perception of institutional style practitioners and practices. This has been particularly damaging for those in mental health and learning disability fields, who for many years were seen as only being able to practise in a hospital setting. It has taken time for fellow professionals and the public to understand and appreciate that the skills nurses acquire in today's training and in their postregistration education can be applied in a wide range of settings. Nurses today are able to adapt and practise in any environment, and the list is long and diverse. They have adjusted their practice to the new environment and, in many cases, to the new employer.

There is no room in the new services for professional jealousy and protectionism over knowledge, skills and expertise, which has occurred in the past. It is now essential at all times for the focal point to be the service user. This is clear whatever document is consulted, be it a government White Paper, literature on clinical governance or a National Service Framework. The future will be about shared and lifelong learning for the entire workforce. This will ensure that essential skills plus knowledge and awareness of the service users' needs and expectations are gained in a setting and environment where professionals learn together.

Some of the current gaps in service provision can be filled by education of existing staff; this does assist useful changes in attitude and in understanding the roles of other team members. It also means that additional resources, while always welcome, are not always necessary to bring about improvements and change in a service. It is false economy to make immediate cuts in staff education budgets when costs need to be cut, and good managers will not fall into this trap. They will recognise that getting staff together in a learning environment is a good investment. The relationships that can and do develop are extremely valuable and cannot be measured in strictly financial terms. For the educationalist, it is a real challenge to change attitudes and get staff to understand other roles; it takes time and requires commitment from all staff. The good signs are when networks start to develop, where improvements in communications start to happen, both formally and informally, and when staff can work together in a well-balanced team.

The introduction and later review of postregistration standards for education and practice (UKCC, 1994, 2001) has set about addressing the educational needs of nurses in the development of specialist practice, particularly for the learning disability nurse in the community. The move to community care, with emphasis on encouraging the client group to adapt from a dependency model of care to total independence where possible, was a real challenge for nurses as well as for their training body. Nursing has survived in this highly competitive and professional arena of care through the efforts of some of the more enlightened and more politically astute nurses, who pioneered new services and developed new and valued roles for the profession. In the authors' opinion, the National Boards for Nursing let learning disability nurses down at this time by the dilatory manner in which they went about updating their education when their practice was changing quickly and radically.

At this time, nurses were being challenged as to whether they had skills that were relevant to the clients' needs in this new service. Many nurses were either reticent or reluctant to come forward and articulate the skills and contribution that they could make and were making. The more enlightened could see that the person with a learning disability often required assistance in basic emotional and physical functions, that could be provided by professional, skilful, educated and caring personnel. This, of course, is the essence of nursing care.

Whenever a minority group struggles for recognition, other dominant and more politically astute groups will argue against that recognition with examples of individual atypical cases. It escaped the notice of many that decision making in small, and often isolated, units needs a registered and professional person who can cope with the depth and breadth of issues that arise. The introduction of PREP belatedly set about addressing the educational needs of all nursing groups and has proved to be an enlightened initiative.

Learning disability nurses have much to celebrate in the new millennium, with many new and exciting projects taking place as community care develops and learning-disabled people become accepted and valued members of our society. Although nurses must not feel complacent, they can feel justifiably proud of the part they have played in these developments. Good examples of this are the nurses who have taken their skills and experience into other services that are not nurse or health led but where their expertise has been invaluable. The health promotion, health education, and well person clinics are other examples of areas where they have made improvements in services.

MAINTAINING STANDARDS

The NMC, which replaced the UKCC, has emphasised a focus on public protection. This is timely and links with the Government's clinical governance agenda, as outlined in *Making a difference* (Department of Health, 1999):

> The Government's plans for quality improvement in the NHS are built around clear national standards, ensuring and monitoring local delivery through clinical governance, supported by professional self-regulation and continuing professional development.
>
> Nurses, midwives and health visitors must play a full part in developing and implementing national service frameworks and clinical governance.

To remain a registered nurse, it is necessary to maintain and update professional knowledge and competence, as outlined in the *Code of professional conduct* (Nursing and Midwifery Council, 2002a). In response to these changes and developments, learning disability nurses have assumed new roles and acquired skills to support and care for their client group in alternative and challenging environments. Practice has expanded and new roles and skills have emerged to facilitate a quality service in the community setting. It is in this area that educationalists have an important role to play in the future of the service, providing support and help for the range of professionals working in the multidisciplinary team.

New skills

New competencies have had to be acquired to enable the service to develop to the standards that are essential. For nurses, this has meant working more flexible hours and arranging their work to meet the needs and preferences of the clients rather than the service or organisation itself. Nurses in learning disability services practise in a range of different settings: from community nurses who carry a caseload through to the nurse working in a home for a small number of people in an ordinary setting outside the NHS. Their client group requires, at times, to have access to a range of services, according to varied and varying needs. In this situation the nurse acts as the broker and liaises with primary health-care colleagues, social workers, specialist health-care services, education, employment and leisure services. The learning disability nurse must often be able to practise a number of therapies, including the management of epilepsy, behavioural psychotherapy, family interventions and grief counselling. An integral part of the nurse's role is facilitating and helping to counterbalance the disempowerment that this minority often faces, to ensure that they have as full and ordinary a life as possible within the constraints and boundaries of their ability and the usual societal constraints.

People with a learning disability are particularly vulnerable to ill-health (Department of Health, 1995). In addition, communication deficits and/or problems with assertiveness can restrict their ability to have their health needs known and, therefore, met (Markwick and Parrish, 1998). The learning disability nurse can assist these individuals to make effective use of the available services.

In the past, risk taking was considered to be outside the nurse's domain. The institutional environment and culture was one in which risk taking was not on the agenda or part of the vocabulary. Risk taking was seen only in terms of the problems it could produce, and the paternalistic, custodial style of service was unable to cope with the consequences if anything went wrong. However, as services developed and moved towards offering a more ordinary living style and natural way of life for service users, there was an expectation that clients could be exposed to the same risks as the average person in the community and could be enabled to cope with managing risk, thereby taking control of their own lives. This new ethos requires support for nurses. Managers and educationalists should work together to produce packages for staff that cover risk taking and risk management in partnership with the people who will be taking the ultimate risk. A policy giving broad guidelines will help staff to feel supported when and if a problem arises.

The path to true community participation and belonging for the learning disabled is long, and steeped in negative attitudes and attempts at oppression and exclusion, albeit in more modern ways recently. There are many people who continue to live segregated lives even within the community, and many tell of greater social restriction now than they experienced within institutional settings. While the 'old days' are gone for good, and rightly so, there is still much work to do in influencing, educating and supporting the public and the other professions to continue to improve the quality of life for this group.

Development and training

The pressure to raise standards, achieve clear and measurable outcomes and ensure that staff have regular opportunities to update their skill base is ongoing and often not accompanied by an increase in resources (Nursing and Midwifery Council, 2002b). This is where the collaboration between services in the important and critical area of multidisciplinary education for staff can be valuable, not only in breaking down barriers between services but also in rationalising educational resources. There is an expectation within central government that new partnership arrangements will take place, and that new markets will emerge; this is accompanied by a desire for links to be made between employers, workforce, education and training providers and validating bodies.

Input from service users

Service providers in health, social and educational services affect both policy development and service development in new areas. There has also been a change in the expectations of both users of learning disability services and their relatives. Within this service, there has been a big improvement in the valuing of the service users; a good example of this is their attendance as full members of planning teams.

Some advocacy groups facilitate training events and offer a valuable and different perspective to professionals and service providers. Such groups have organised training events for members of the multidisciplinary team and demonstrated a positive outcome and rationale for service user involvement. There have also been opportunities for service users to join education, curriculum planning and delivery groups; in the authors' experience, this has been particularly beneficial. This, in turn, has caused service providers to consider the issue of appropriate remuneration and support for service users who participate in planning and teaching. In many universities these days, it is not uncommon for people with learning disabilities to be employed as part-time or visiting lecturers and to be entitled to all the benefits one would expect, including salary and entitlements to access the hallowed senior common room.

James Newland and a team of six service users from an advocacy project are now participating in both higher and further education planning and provision. They report that they enjoy the experience themselves and have received training to enable them to develop their skills. The students benefit from the experience and value the input. The sessions are designed to avoid possible tokenism by requiring James and his colleagues to seek out views of users and carers in the locality and represent them as well as their own views. There will always be a problem in truly being able to engage with people with the most severe and profound learning disability, but this has to be a step in the right direction.

Interagency cooperation

In any agenda for change, educational opportunities must cover both issues relating to organisational changes, and their implications, and the individual's professional updating. For education to play a full and effective part in the new user-led services, there must be commitment from managers and staff and adequate resources. Interagency cooperation is not new for the learning disability workforce, where commitment and collaboration between professionals have ensured a fair deal for many service users and their relatives, even when this has meant bending the rules and taking risks.

Educationalists can help to develop this cooperation by working with staff at senior levels to ensure that prejudices and unhelpful barriers are broken down. Often the problem among professionals is the complete lack of understanding of their colleagues' role, skill-base and knowledge. Opportunities for staff to get together in a stress-free and non-challenging environment to share experiences and values will help to reduce barriers. Thompson (2001) pointed out that these barriers form part of the challenge associated with progress in interprofessional training in the area of learning disability services. This phenomenon is well researched (Brown and Thompson, 1988; Shaw, 1993; Thompson and Mathias, 1998). Thompson (2001) highlights some of the barriers:

- agency failure to release appropriate staff for training
- inadequate financial backing for relevant training
- lack of empathy and understanding between contributing agencies
- insufficient involvement of service users and carers in the design of training programmes
- poor commitment to joint training by statutory bodies and senior management.

Professional updating It is with this backdrop in mind that nurses must set about facilitating improved education and professional updating. Nursing bodies are looking at the educational needs of all nurses and at moving further into higher education. Lifelong learning has become a term often heard in education and nursing, following the publication of the Dearing report on higher education (National Committee of Inquiry into Higher Education, 1997). The principle was that all individuals must take responsibility for their own development, creating a learning organisation and thereby a learning society. The report holds that people from all walks of life will continue with training and education in order to keep abreast of rapid change: in the world, at work and in their lives.

The overt message in the report is that we all need to learn throughout our lives. A learning disability nurse will be considering the constant training, development and updating that will be needed to maintain knowledge and nursing expertise in rapidly changing and developing community services for people with a disability. Lifelong learning (Thomson, 2002) can present itself in many different ways, ranging from a formal course to a study day or to a session spent with a colleague who imparts some of their expertise.

Regardless of the means adopted, gaining knowledge from any source will increase self-confidence and credibility among colleagues, as well as maintaining personal esteem. What is important about education is not what you learn but how it changes you and your practice.

This is an era in which all registered nurses, midwives and health visitors have to be responsible for their own learning and professional development, and that of others, irrespective of their own role or the service in which they work, be that the NHS, county council or the private sector. The mandatory requirements for PREP place lifelong learning firmly on the agenda so that nurses can ensure that their own practice is contemporary at all times. PREP also sets and maintains a professional standard that is an important factor in the multidisciplinary team. Individual nurses, through PREP, will maintain and improve the quality of their practice, as well as develop their standards through deeper insight and understanding.

Thomson (2002) explains that the study days in PREP can be interpreted broadly and creatively. Some nurses will organise for themselves attendance at conferences, workshops or study days for 5 days regardless of whether this meets their individual learning needs or not. This is not what the spirit of PREP is about; it is about encouraging the development of practice and skills at a level and pace that suits the individual and current need. Five days equates to about 35 hours of study, which is open to broad interpretation, and individual nurses should let PREP help them meet their own needs. This part of the PREP process is often overlooked as nurses strive to achieve their 5 update days and focus on adding certificates to their portfolio. For true learning and development to take place nurses should establish:

- why they choose to study what they do
- how they bring that back to the practice arena
- how they evaluate the positive impact.

Simply ticking the box and collecting the certificate is not what the process is fundamentally about. Study can be interpreted as:

- a workshop or study day
- reading
- a focussed visit to another area of practice with objectives to achieve upon the nurse's return
- time spent with another practitioner with different skills and expertise to one's own
- the use of distance learning material
- a taught course
- a formal professional debate.

As an example, a nurse may attend a conference on epilepsy and learn much about clients' behaviour and the value of some of the modern medications, leaving the conference with a better and updated knowledge base. It is then up to the nurse to use this knowledge and apply it to practice in the most appropriate way for the benefit of the client group, and to share this new information with colleagues. Thomson goes on to suggest that an individual may, following the experience at the conference, feel that some time could be valuably spent at a library on a focused literature search on this aspect of care. She points out that active note taking and reading are a valid updating activity provided that the learning is applied to practice. The literature search may produce questions and issues that could be answered by organising some time with a clinical nurse specialist in epilepsy so that the theoretical studies can be supplemented with the added benefit of another nurse's experience.

Consequently, a single activity that does not take up the full 5 days may nevertheless generate points to be explored with other health workers, or a parent or relative of a client, ethical issues to be pursued and further reading to do. This can quickly develop into 35 hours and all that is needed is to make some relevant notes and confirm what you intend to do with your new learning.

Boxes 8.1 and 8.2 describe two approaches to PREP, which illustrate this point. Which of these nurses would you employ or want as a member of your team? Clearly these examples are given to show a polarisation of attitudes, but do not think these attitudes do not exist, because they do. Many people do not fully appreciate the philosophy of PREP and see it as a box-ticking exercise. If it is to be real it must be much more.

Box 8.1	**John Webster, a qualified nurse**

John Webster is a qualified nurse with over 5 years' experience. He has been working with the same client group for some years and he feels that he has acquired all the necessary skills to discharge his duties appropriately. John is aware that his registration is due for renewal in the next few months and he is keen to ensure that his portfolio is up to date with the appropriate evidence of development and learning. He can identify 4 days' worth of training through 1- and 2-day courses he has been on and he has put the certificates in his folder in readiness. They fit in his folder in a specific divider marked 'personal/professional development certificates' and only certificates are filed here. John sees no reason to record a rationale for course choice or application of the learning in the practice area. He feels that that would only be necessary if he was not doing formal courses and getting the all-important certificate to prove it. He feels confident that he would impress the NMC if they audited his folder and he feels positive about the folder being an asset when he comes to look for a new job in the future. John has one more day's study to find before he can rest easy about his continued status as a Registered Nurse. He looks through the available literature on courses and is attracted to a 1-day seminar on challenging behaviour. But the seminar is some distance away, starts early and does not specifically say that there is a certificate of attendance. Although it might be useful for his practice, John rejects the seminar. Instead he opts for a 1-day course on policy and practice, which is very similar to a course he has done previously. He knows there is a certificate of attendance as it is an internal course and he knows that there is no requirement for him to do anything more than attend for the day to achieve what he needs. He applies for a place, gets his certificate and adds it to his folder.

| Box 8.2 | **Emily Jones, a newly qualified nurse** |

Emily Jones is a newly qualified nurse who is working within a health setting for people with severe and profound learning disabilities. She has developed a keen interest in the physical health of people who cannot communicate through traditional means. She works with a number of people who are vulnerable to health challenges and who are unable to communicate any detail of how they feel or what their specific needs are. She identifies, through supervision with her manager, that there is a need to develop a robust system of physical health checks for at least four of the residents. Up to now, they have relied on ad hoc checks when residents' behaviour changes indicated that a problem may be occurring. She begins with a literature search to identify what has been learnt already. The work is done during 1 or 2 hours that she is able to make available either in work time or in her own time. This uncovers helpful information about projects that have been piloted and evaluated, and tools that have been tried and tested. She prepares a paper for her team outlining what she has read and condensing the relevant facts into an accessible form. She presents it at a team meeting and most of the team are very excited by the proposal. One member of staff is cynical and cannot see a reason to change. In supervision, the health check project is discussed and refined and the next stage is planned. In addition, they begin to explore the member of staff's opposition and methods Emily might adopt to persuade him. She begins to do some additional work around influence and change management in addition to launching, for two residents, the health check system that had been chosen. The project identifies that one resident has a urinary tract infection and the other has a degenerative sight problem that had not been previously identified. Appropriate measures are taken to address the issues and the process is broadened to all other residents. Emily continues to work with the cynical member of staff and takes trouble to show the positive results in order to persuade and involve him. The process is slow but measurable. In supervision, the process is monitored and Emily begins to record the process in her portfolio, including the outcomes, impact on the clients, the service and the team. She considers writing this up for a professional journal.

The lifelong learning model and the approach taken by PREP give a useful framework that could easily be applied to the non-nursing professions who work with people with a learning disability.

Thomson (2002) suggests that teaching and learning for professional updating can be streamlined and focussed on the individual's clinical area of practice. In learning disability services, this may be in a wide variety of settings and across a number of different agencies. Whatever the practice arena, it is imperative that there is good quality leadership and the newly appointed nurse consultants and modern matrons can provide the impetus for this.

The Government has recognised that the level of skills, training and qualification in the learning disability workforce needs to be raised, and to encourage progress in this area have from April 2001 introduced a Learning Disability Awards Framework. This fits comfortably into existing qualification structures and provides a recognised route to qualification and career progression for care workers in the services. Initially, there have been some concerns about the effects this might have on recruitment and retention of staff, given the intensity and standard of the course; while the principle is sound, it would seem that there is scope for formal evaluation.

Many managers have been released from their service to attend senior management courses on leadership development and understanding. Yet they can still find it hard to realise that, whatever managers do and however effective they think they are, the organisation they work in is only as good as the staff. Generally, managers do not give this facet of their responsibility enough priority and yet it is the basis of good management thinking and the theme of so many management courses. It is to be hoped that, in the future development and organisation of services for people with a learning disability, managers in all service provision situations will come to realise this and also see the value of continuing education and multidisciplinary working. A vehicle for this will be the recently reconfigured Workforce Education and Development Confederations, who are charged with commissioning educational programmes and taking the Government's health and social care agenda forward.

REFLECTIVE PRACTICE

It is an interesting exercise to sit with colleagues and reflect on the changes that have taken place in your area of practice over the past year or two. Just spend some time looking at the recent publications, for example from the NMC and the Royal College of Nursing, to get an insight into how quickly and radically things change and how important it is to be in tune and up to date with these changes. Reflective practice is a system that all nurses contribute to and that helps all nurses to keep up to date. Some services use journal clubs or regular monthly lunchtime sessions where team members take turns to share with others the latest professional news. The ability to keep abreast of change also depends on lifelong learning, which ensures you remain flexible and open, questioning and able to evaluate a challenge.

Reflective practice is more common now than ever before, and many professions could learn from the reflective culture that is evident within learning disability nursing. However, we can all benefit from more structured opportunities for reflection, and assisted reflection either in groups or in one-to-one sessions can be extremely useful. Nurses can be complacent regarding reflection and may think, for example, that it can be done equally well simply by thinking about work issues during daily journeys. Learning is an active process; it works best when it is planned and it requires thoughts to be organised. Formal reflection can take this process to new depths and can really have a positive impact on practice. Reflective teams are being developed. Organisations, through clinical governance, are becoming familiar with concepts such as openness and a learning culture. This all makes the future an exciting place full of challenge and opportunity.

CONCLUSIONS In *Valuing people* (Department of Health, 2001), the Government maintained that services need a firm value base and clear objectives in order to improve the lives of people with learning disabilities. If the strategy is to succeed, there needs to be a strong commitment nationally and locally to upholding individual legal and civil rights and promoting independence, choice and inclusion. Each individual should have the required support and opportunity to be the person he or she wants to be. Learning disability nurses have key parts to play in the development of these new services. Their skills, knowledge and experience are a valuable asset, as is their ability to work in a multidisciplinary team and across organisational boundaries.

Learning disability nurses are unique in respect of their professional accountability to the NMC and for maintaining their clinical competence as outlined in the *Code of professional conduct* (Nursing and Midwifery Council, 2002a) and *Making a difference* (Department of Health, 1999). For this strategy to be successful, managers and education providers have to ensure that the principles of lifelong learning are established and followed within their services. Workforce Education and Development Confederations have a crucial part to play in this as they must ensure that educational programmes are available to all professional groups, are contemporary and are of a high quality.

The Government's strategic intentions for nursing, midwifery and health visiting and its commitment to strengthen and to maximise their contribution to the NHS is very clearly spelt out (Department of Health, 1999). One of the key points in Chapter 1 of *Making a difference* (Department of Health, 1999) is a good point to conclude this chapter. 'Nurses, Midwives and Health Visitors are vital to the NHS, and to the nation: they make a real difference to people's lives. People trust them, and have confidence in them. People value what they do. So does the Government.'

ACKNOWLEDGE-MENTS The authors wish to acknowledge the help and assistance of Sally Thomson and Lesley Styring in the preparation of this chapter.

REFERENCES

Birchenall P, Parrish A 1997 Learning disability nursing and primary healthcare. British Journal of Nursing 6(2): 92–98

Brown J, Thompson A R 1998 Quality and care: a positive approach to the future. Royal College of Nursing/Mental Handicap Nurses Association, London

Department of Health 1995 Health of the nation for people with learning disabilities. HMSO, London

Department of Health 1999 Making a difference. Strengthening the nursing, midwifery and health visiting contribution to health and healthcare. The Stationery Office, London

Department of Health 2001 Valuing people: a new strategy for learning disability for the 21st century. The Stationery Office, London

Markwick A, Parrish A 1998 Equity and access to healthcare for women with learning disabilities. British Journal of Nursing 7(2): 92–96

National Committee of Inquiry into Higher Education 1997 The Dearing report: Higher Education in the Learning Society. HMSO London

Nursing and Midwifery Council 2002a Code of professional conduct. NMC, London

Nursing and Midwifery Council 2002b NMC News, Spring Number 1. NMC, London

Parrish A 2002 Prison health care—who needs a nurse? Nursing Management 8(8): 6–9

Pearce L 2001 Don't stop now. Nursing Standard 16(2): 14

Shaw I 1993 The politics of inter-professional training—lessons for learning disability. Journal of Inter-Professional Care 7(3): ??

Thompson T 2001 Challenges and opportunities in education and training. In: Sines D, Appleby F, Raymond E (eds) Community health care nursing, 2nd edn. Blackwell Science, Oxford

Thompson T, Mathias P 1998 Standards and learning disability, 2nd edn. Baillière Tindall, London

Thomson S 2002 Enhancing practice through education. In: Norman A, Parrish A (eds) Prison nursing. Blackwell Science, Oxford, pp 261–272

UKCC 1992 Code of professional practice. UKCC, London

UKCC 1993 The Council's position concerning a period of support and preceptorship: implementation of the post-registration and practice project (PREPP) (Registrar's Letter 1/1993). UKCC, London

UKCC 1994 Standards for education and practice following registration: the future of professional practice. UKCC, London

UKCC 2001 Standards of specialist education and practice (Registrar's letter 11/2001). UKCC, London

Planning and monitoring of care

Brian McGinnis

This chapter is concerned with the effects that current changes in care have on the individual person with learning difficulties. Using examples, it describes the problems that can occur when planning and theory lose touch with the actual individuals affected. The issues of consultation and monitoring are discussed as vital aspects of developing and assessing plans over time. Finally, the incorporation of flexibility into plans is considered in order to help the service user to find their own version of happiness.

THE MOVE TO COMMUNITY CARE Earlier chapters have discussed the change in thinking behind care for those with learning disabilities over the last 100 years. Every time a change in policy is implemented it affects individual vulnerable people. One such person is Charles, who started off in a small, by NHS standards, group of 15 children (Box 9.1). The changes imposed on Charles are an example of planning for people rather than with them.

Box 9.1	Charles's first care home

> The unit in which Charles lived was small by NHS standards, but large by ordinary living standards. He was part of a group of 15 children who had once slept on an open ward, but who now had curtained cubicles and thus a certain amount of privacy. The children shared a combined dining room and play area. The unit was in fairly self-contained grounds but within pushing distance of local shops, churches and leisure facilities; it was also within easy reach of the volunteers of various ages who came in from the local community. 'Separate but not isolated' would have been a good description.

The first change was implemented when Charles was 13 years old. The parents of the 15 children were gathered together and it was explained that 15 was a 'bad' number and five was a 'good' number; therefore, all the children would have homes for life in houses with five residents (Box 9.2). It was also explained that with community care the children would be able to visit the local community, spend their money in the local shops, get to know the local people and hold conversations with their neighbours. Charles's parents were rather puzzled by all this and upset, not because they were puzzled but because they saw Charles losing his security. Charles had never held a conversation with anyone and was most unlikely ever to do so; he had no concept of the relationship between money and goods. However, he was already visiting the local shops and getting to know local people, and he was well known in return. Charles's parents, fairly or unfairly, drew the conclusion that those who were planning the move did not know Charles, and if they did not know Charles they were not well placed to plan for Charles—however sound their planning principles. Regardless of this, Charles was moved.

Box 9.2	**Charles's second care home**

In due course Charles was moved to quite a nice house in quite a nice area, with four other children with whom he had nothing much in common except some compatibility of needs. The chosen neighbourhood was not wholly convenient for Charles's parents, but houses had to be bought where houses were available. In the new neighbourhood, Charles, still silent, visited local shops, became known to local people but rather lost out on volunteer visitors because such visiting was seen as not wholly consistent with ordinary living.

Five years passed and Charles became an adult, a change in status that, although inevitable, apparently had not been anticipated. It was decreed that houses dedicated to children should not be used by adults, although in ordinary life mixed age use and growing up into adulthood in the same house are actually not uncommon. So, in time, Charles was moved again (Box 9.3), not for his own sake but to ensure that his 'home for life' was available for some other children. Before long Charles was on the move again—back eventually, strangely enough, to the non-community care site from which he had been moved when community care came on the scene (Box 9.4).

Box 9.3	**Charles must leave his children's placement**

Charles was moved again to live in a different house with different people in a different area, a temporary move to free up his 'child's' place as he was now 18 years old. Another chance to visit, silently, local shops, get to be known by local people, but not to spend pocket money since adults do not get pocket money. They get a personal allowance.

Charles's final home

Before long Charles was on the move again. He was returned to the non-community care site from which he had been moved when community care came on the scene. He shares with four other people and visits (still silent) the same local shops he had visited as a child and gets to be known by those who meet him. Volunteer visitors no longer exist, so he tends to meet fewer people than he did when he first lived on the site.

While this is a 'case' example that combines features of several different personal stories, it is an example of planning for people, or rather making plans and then fitting people into them, rather than planning with them. Charles was never consulted in any way.

PRINCIPLES VERSUS PEOPLE

At the time of writing, Joint Investment Plans for people with learning disabilities are at various stages of production (these were due in April 2001). Within some plans that were started late enough to reflect the White Paper *Valuing people* (Department of Health, 2001), the beginning of a process of converting existing processes into the required new processes can be seen. This is particularly welcome in person-centred planning, which is intended to be more than just a token form of personal planning. No doubt, there were and are paper ambitions for Charles, but those paper ambitions seem not to have had any particular bearing on the major changes in his life. Nor did anyone seem to see any inconsistency between having written goals for some of the minutiae of daily life, while deciding quite separately for him where he lived, who he lived with and the degree of continuity or discontinuity in contact with family or friends or acquaintances.

In what sense would the story of Charles have differed if person-centred planning, as the White Paper envisages it, had been in place? It is not sufficient to be content with a different set of papers and new training courses on how to complete the new papers. Unless what actually happens is radically reorientated, redesigning the formal process, these moves have, like 'the flowers that bloom in the Spring', nothing to do with the case (to re-use W S Gilbert).

If this radical interpretation of person-centred planning had been implemented for Charles, it would have ensured several important issues were acknowledged and acted upon:

- Who and what were important in Charles's life would be clearly acknowledged, and maintaining and improving those valued things would be a priority.
- There would be a practical ambition to build up his circle of friends.
- A means would be established for determining with Charles his short- and long-term aspirations. In other words, a communication

passport would be established, a genuine process of 'nothing for Charles without Charles', involving those closest to him in this very personal dialogue. A system of 'We decide; he suffers the consequences; you keep quiet' represents service-centred planning and is the complete antithesis of person-centred planning.

- The perceptions of the staff who worked most closely with Charles would be taken on board so that they, he and Charles's family are masters and not servants of the system that provides for him.
- It would be agreed that Charles will move if, and only if, that particular move is one he wants to make, is in his best interests and is right for him personally at that particular time.
- Principles should be subjugated to person, to the extent that 'We don't do that sort of thing here' becomes 'We don't usually do that sort of thing here, but since that is what you want, it will be done'.

This is radical thinking; if it had happened 15 years ago, it might have meant Charles staying where he was. That, in turn, might have meant the unit manager telling the service manager in the local agency that closing the unit was not acceptable. The message would be passed effectively up the line, from the local agency to the district, the region and, finally, the central government, that the declared goal of closing all such units was not achievable. Safe person-centred planning has existed for years: safe in the sense of marginal. Major issues have been determined by service principles, the daily routines by service practice and convenience, and only the fringe decisions by person-centred planning. As St Augustine found with virtue, which he wanted to practise but not whole-heartedly and not yet, you cannot have person-centred planning as an add-on, a coat of paint on the front door to mislead the customers.

My favourite St Francis (of Assissi) story is of the two warring armies, the Emperor, no less, on one side, about to engage in battle; St Francis intervened to tell them they would have to fight somewhere else because a bird was nesting in a bush in the middle of the battlefield. It is possible to conceive of a person-centred plan being stymied by lack of resources. It is not acceptable for a person-centred plan to be stymied by service principles. If principles take pride of place, then what is happening is not person-centred planning, it is service-centred planning masquerading as person-centred planning.

Finding a compromise Charles's state of health is such that he is probably not going to be moved again, although there are periodic re-runs of the principled arguments that led to his initial move 15 years previously. He is, therefore, like so many others, in a place that was not arrived at in discussion with him and with people he did not choose as his companions. The person-centred parts of Charles's life are vulnerable to all the constraints that result from limited and not wholly predictable cash resources. Staff sickness, staff training, recruitment and retention difficulties could all impinge on his plan: saying 'hydrotherapy' in the plan does not guarantee that there will be hydrotherapy. Audit in most services regularly identifies a gap between goals and achievements, but that gap is not necessarily anyone's fault.

We need to face the challenge that person-centred planning can be merely a grandiose dream with no real impact on reality. While person-centred minutiae do not compensate for all the big decisions being taken on a quite different basis, the opposite is also true. Big changes in people's lives are, for most people, not all that common; and the chance every decade or so to be partner in a big decision is no great consolation for having your daily life for 10-year stretches determined by the system and the system's lack of resources. Person-centred planning is now possible in the daily lives of people for whom big negotiated change is a long way off.

There are major policy choices to be made in this period following *Valuing people* (Department of Health, 2001). One option is to cling to the outmoded belief that service models do hold the answer—a belief about which the White Paper is part-cynical and part-ambivalent. That option concentrates on closing the hospitals, closing the NHS campuses and, in due course, closing the residential homes; this will result in supported living (however defined) and family placements becoming the norm. In other words, the energy goes into another round of resettlement, and resettlement tends to be an uneasy compromise between numbers and principles and people. Lorna Wing's critique of part of the Darenth Park resettlement rankled because she asked awkward questions about what was actually happening in a process where numbers did loom rather large (Wing, 1989).

As the National Development Team (1988) noted in its report on Calderstones and Brockhall, there is a serious risk that, if putting people somewhere else is the outcome measure, the quality of the lives of those not yet moved may actually deteriorate. Resettlement is often seen as a more acceptable performance indicator than personal happiness. Even before *Valuing people* (Department of Health, 2001), there were local authorities saying 'We don't do residential care any more'. Now there could be many more celebrating home closures as the measure of success in fulfilling White Paper ambitions.

TAKING PERSON-CENTRED PLANNING SERIOUSLY

If person-centred planning is to be taken seriously, it does not allow this resettlement approach. Person-centred planning takes five people living in a residential home as five individuals with histories, relationships, ambitions, dreams and futures, and it addresses what those five individuals want and need here and now and in the longer term. There is nothing so very strange in this approach. Most of us have a constant process of experiment and adjustment built around a stable personal core agenda of earning a living and staying passably healthy and out of trouble. We rearrange the furniture, build a rockery, try a new restaurant, get to know a new neighbour, sign on at the gym, experiment with tofu as an alternative food, throw out the seashell vase from Guernsey.

Incessant change is more attractive only for a minority; however, even those with a strong desire for familiarity and continuity find enough things not quite right to result in regular review and revision. That may be a more appropriate and realistic approach than a dominant resettlement agenda for most people with learning disabilities most of the time. One argument for being wary of resettlement is the recognition that it is quite possible to move people to new situations only to recreate all the disadvantages of the old situation. A family placement or supported living placement may be just as institutional as a large institution—without the excuses of size and numbers.

Opportunity mapping

How then would person-centred planning be applied to Charles's current circumstances if the prospect of a further move is remote?

The starting point might be mapping Charles's *support network*—relatives, friends, staff who know him well—and examining how these contacts could be made easier. Are there transport problems? Could the shift system be better designed to give Charles time with those staff members he really likes? Are there more possibilities for shared events and celebrations? In L'Arche (Spink, 1990; see also Ch. 2 for a discussion of the L'Arche communities), something significant is always being celebrated, whether for core members, families or assistants. The celebrations are inclusive and sensitive. As Mary said, 'I like visitors; and I like it when they go'.

The next question would be whether there are possibilities to *extend this network*? Is a personal citizen advocate an option, and if so what would their role be? Does Charles have funds for a sessional supporter if staff resources do not allow as many local visits as Charles would like? Are there elderly relatives who would like to visit but find the journey awkward? Is it really unacceptable for Charles to be involved with staff's families, social networks and special occasions?

The next step would be *pleasure*: to map, with those who know Charles, what Charles most and least enjoys. What might he enjoy if he had the opportunity? Some things are quite simple. Charles thought the Morris dancers were hilarious, and that is worth trying again.

It would also add another dimension to the old socialisation convention of visiting the pub so that the staff can have a drink (if local rules allow drinking on duty). Others, like the flight in the aeroplane, are not simple but for a number of people can provide the memory of a lifetime. Six years on, one man still points to the sky and points to himself when the plane goes overhead.

Opportunity mapping necessarily includes seeking out *local resources*: the folk club; the keep fit class; the activities and worship in a local church; the Woman's Institute, Townswomen's Guild or Woman's Rural; the annual carnival; the pantomime, on stage or in the audience. Charles likes music but if he is not very well, a musician coming in to play the guitar and sing might have the edge on the theatre, where the performance time might be too long. All these activities will require personnel support: volunteers, relatives, friends and staff. Charles may need stesolid but seldom does; stesolid-centred planning is not the same as person-centred planning.

Record keeping Audit does tend these days to take personal plans into account, even though much of audit is of service systems and not directly of personal happiness. However, assuming some continuity of staffing, unit staff will know someone like Charles as a person, whereas senior management may not. Just as residential units commonly have photographs of staff and a brief description to help residents and visitors know who is who, they must also have individual personal records of residents. Managers and staff should have a photograph and a brief personal profile of each resident—to capture and communicate something of the person that those closer to them know.

This part of record keeping should include positive features (Box 9.5). Planning does also include risk assessment, which necessarily includes the negatives of people's lives.

Box 9.5	**A brief personal profile**
	Charles has flexion deformities of all four limbs, scoliosis, epilepsy, is doubly incontinent and mute; he has difficulties in swallowing and resists taking liquids. Charles has a sense of humour, a delightful smile, a great enjoyment of people (in small quantities) and a love for classical music. He has a sweet tooth.

Who makes decisions? There is a long, though not an honourable, tradition of service planning being done by those sufficiently remote from service users to know nothing of them as people, and individual planning being done by those who have a very short time to pick up from assessment what others know already from long experience. Indeed, remoteness and ignorance have been paraded as the virtues of independence and fresh insight, whereas those who know the person well are seen as having acquired a blinkered view and as being at risk of judging their own interests and not the person's best interests.

True person-centred planning can only be done by or in consultation with those who know the person. If the person does not communicate, that implies knowing them well. The 'Oh that's the one with the red hair, isn't it?' approach to assessment and planning will not deliver person-centred planning. Nor will service planning that is detached from person-centred planning and over-rules the latter.

For example, in one service, the senior manager could introduce a visitor to staff, though not to service users, but was rather thrown when a member of staff asked him who he was. In a different service, the senior manager knew every member of staff and every service user not only by name but by current concerns and recent achievements: and they all knew him. When the Trust Board or the Local Authority takes a decision affecting people's lives, it should be briefed by those who know the people as people and should have at least some positive pen portraits of those people. 'We need to relocate five people in order to make the most cost-efficient use of buildings, and relatives have been informed—net savings £40 000' does sound rather different as a decision from 'One of those who would have to move is Charles, who has had one move already this year and has just settled and begun to seem at home. He now smiles at visitors instead of looking apprehensive.'

Focussing on the individual

Focussing on the individual is easier for a case worker is than it is for a planner. The planner faces a number of difficulties:

- nobody has yet explained convincingly how you convert several hundred individual plans into a service plan
- the greater the reliance on individual satisfaction as an outcome measure, the greater the risk of failure—because individual wishes have been misread or individual wishes have changed
- it is difficult to work with someone who is being asked to assess the potential benefits of something they have never experienced
- relying on well-informed third parties is legitimate where there are communication and understanding barriers; but what if the various third parties disagree on best interests?
- planning is not always about accessing what already is; it may be about creating something new: this is easier to achieve with a meal or visit but less easy for a post or service.

The philosophy underlying person-centred planning is trying to capture for other people what we spend our lives trying to capture for ourselves. Those who can exercise their choices continually question and change their minds. What do I know? What do I value? What do I want to try out? What risks am I willing to take? What price am I willing to pay? What am I trying to achieve? How do I know I have 'arrived'? I will seek information and I will listen to advice, but this is at the end of the day about me and for me, and I am the only one who can judge whether it was all worthwhile.

In seeking our own welfare, we may be willing to compromise in the interests of others, to keep the good opinion of those we value or because we recognise that unfulfilled dreams are part of life. Unless we have major personality problems, we do not live our lives by other people's standards, for other people's convenience or to fulfil other people's planning goals. We even want to make our own mistakes, and we derive no lasting satisfaction from making other people's mistakes.

ADVOCACY: TALKING AND LISTENING

The language of self-advocacy very easily lapses into a discussion of verbalisation. Self-advocacy should be a matter of creating opportunity and support for people to formulate mentally their own opinions, to express those opinions verbally and to assert the moral right to be heard. Self-advocacy can extend, though not always successfully, from being the private expression of personal views about personal interests to being the very public expression of collective views about collective interests. It can also, though less commonly, become the private or public expression of personal views about the personal interests of a third party, who is not speaking. In this context, reading and writing are not hugely important, but verbal ability is.

It is a perfectly legitimate shift from strictly self-advocacy to group advocacy and advocacy for others and it is legitimate for service planners to listen to it. A service planner wishing to benefit from the advocacy of a person or group to get as close as possible to the unvocalised wishes of another should be aware of three factors:

- All humans communicate and there needs to be investment in establishing how the person at the centre communicates, and in supporting consistent communication and consistent interpretation of that communication.
- There should be at least one person who is close enough to and often enough with the person at the centre to become a credible translator. In the family setting, this may be a parent and/or a sibling. In a service setting, it may be a key worker, or it may be a volunteer or advocate who is regularly able to be with the person.

- It is good to have more than one person as an expert translator, for example a circle of friends. This is both because different people tend to hear different things and because the communication of the person at the centre may actually vary between different audiences and different settings. It is also because some of this translation work is a little speculative, and it is as well to be cautious about the translator who is always quite 'certain' what somebody without words is saying.

A good example is that of Joey Deacon from St Lawrence's, where one person with a learning disability spoke, from a shared experience, for the interests of another person with a learning disability (Deacon, 1977). Joey could speak but the problem was that most people could not clearly understand what he was saying. The whole process that produced Joey's story was dependent not on the intermediary being able to talk but on the intermediary being able and willing to *listen.* In addition, all three men involved in the process lived together and closely shared a common experience.

The service/opportunity planner who uses a verbal self-advocate or self-advocacy group to understand the interests and wishes of someone who does not use words needs to be aware of how much listening and shared experience underlies what is being said. The messages may still be legitimate without much listening or shared experience, but only at the level of service principles, not at the level of person-centred planning.

A SHARED JOURNEY? The very useful L'Arche expression 'Walking with' can be linked with the Native American saying about walking in another man's moccasins before you judge that man. L'Arche communities around the world put great stress on accompaniment and walking with, because sharing someone's daily journey with them inevitably helps understanding. If you are close to someone and listening to them, you stand a much better chance of translating accurately. 'Walking with' requires skill and concentration as well as positioning: it is possible to share a park bench, a view and a conversation, but to be mutually uncomprehending.

People who work in services are thoroughly, and properly, grounded in the principle of 'do as you would be done by', but this should be tempered by remembering that this is only a tentative starting point for making a judgement about someone else's interests. It is fairly safe to assume that nobody wants to be cold, thirsty, hungry or inappropriately dressed for the occasion and so on; however, the higher one moves up the Maslow hierarchy, the more choices differ, and the less personal choices can be confidently projected onto others. We have all seen a companion clearly enjoying an outing and very clear in their own mind that their silent partner is equally enjoying it, when the partner's body language says otherwise. So personal preferences can be a sound starting point for trying something, but a trial is, by definition, something of which the outcome is uncertain.

That leads on to the sensitive issue of what is age appropriate, and whether being age appropriate actually matters. In the context of learning disability, the sensitivity stems from the discredited notions of 'mental age' and 'perpetual children'. There is a natural reluctance to allow people to behave in ways that could create or confirm prejudice against them. Some aspects of this reflect basic common sense. It is not uncommon for a small child, in an emergency, to go to the toilet with parental help in a rather public way. This is not appropriate for an older person. It is not uncommon for small children to do without clothes when the mood takes them. Older people cannot be allowed that discretion, whether they want it or not. However, adults do have soft toys or comfort objects; adults do at times indulge in quite childish behaviour, even when they have substantial adult resources and easy access to activities more conventionally associated with adults.

It is not right to be narrow minded about what is age appropriate so that people are denied meaningful opportunities in the absence of any acceptable alternatives. Charles in his teens might have been more age appropriately occupied with strobe lighting at a disco than with bubble tubes and a water bed, but he liked the Snoezelen room whereas the strobe lighting would have brought on fits. Sandra liked to carry around her family photo album and share it with visitors, which most non-disabled women of her age would not have done. However, women of her age quite commonly carry in a handbag or wallet photos of boy friend, husband or children, which they are keen to share.

Once again, there is nothing wrong with having principles in service planning, but the relevance of the principle to the person must be considered and whether the person is the beneficiary or the victim of the principle.

SIGNING THE CONTRACT

The idea of a contract causes some difficulties in learning disability services. First, a contract is normally an agreement between two parties, with obligations on both sides; and not everybody with a learning disability would be considered competent to sign their side of the agreement. Second, there is a tradition of reluctance to commit to more than best endeavours when so many things might change that would make a promise difficult to keep. Nevertheless, there is much to be said for giving people such assurances as are possible about what is going to happen for them. This is what was envisaged in the Griffiths (1988) report: care assessments would be reflected in care plans, and the service user would have a copy of the care plan, including, it was hoped, a note on those things that were justified and intended but not yet deliverable.

A support or care contract will be a written record of who will be doing what, when they will be doing it, what the purpose is, what if anything it will cost and when the arrangements will be reviewed. It will also give a contact person with whom to discuss any problems, and it will explain the complaints process. In situations and with people where agreements on both sides are possible, there could be a mutual contract—as with someone competent to sign up to a tenancy agreement in which the tenant has obligations. In other cases, the contract will explain for the benefit of relatives or advocates the circumstances in which contract arrangements might need to be reviewed out of sequence.

The strongest argument for this degree of formality is that so often there is misunderstanding about what has been agreed informally. Within the last year, the following complaints have been made to me:

- the guarantee of a home for life has been broken
- a guaranteed day service has been withdrawn
- other people with incompatible needs have been introduced into the home without consultation, despite promises to the contrary
- staff have not acquired the skills promised at signing
- a holiday had been promised but not delivered
- therapy had been scheduled but not provided
- respite promises had been broken.

None of these things had been written down, and in each case the relative or advocate had been convinced that promises had been made while the service manager was equally clear that promises had not been made.

The care/support contract should guarantee the basics, subject to review, and the care/support plan should set out the detail within the framework of the contract. This detail is likely to be subject to more frequent review and is likely to be at greater risk of unplanned change because of staffing or other difficulties. If a staff member calls in sick, and nobody else can provide quite the same support, then plans have to be changed despite everybody's best endeavours.

The provision of a *support contract* is illustrated in Box 9.6, which describes the type of provision that might be outlined for someone like Margaret: living at home with family and having high support needs and uncertain health.

| Box 9.6 | A support contract |

Margaret lives at home with her family. She has high support needs, and rather uncertain health.

Miss Margaret Mead of .... [address]

Mother: Mrs Ruth Mead

On behalf of ..... agency/authority), I undertake that a chairlift will be provided and installed for Margaret's use on 31 May 2001 (or such other date as is agreed with Mrs Mead). The costs will be met in full by this agency/authority.

A day service on weekdays throughout the year will be available at the ..... Centre, and transport for Margaret from her home to the Centre and back will be provided. Normal pick up time at Margaret's home will be 9.30 a.m., and Margaret will normally be home again by 5 p.m. Should any change in these arrangements be necessary, we will endeavour to give at least 24 hours notice. No charges will be made for Centre attendance or for transport.

A two day/one night short-term break at ..... will be scheduled for Margaret each calendar month on days to be agreed between the unit and Mrs Mead. Transport will be arranged between the unit and Margaret's home or the unit and the Centre, as appropriate. No charges will be made for these services. Should any changes be needed in planned breaks, Mrs Mead will be notified at least 48 hours in advance and new dates will be negotiated.

Mrs Mead has agreed to give at least three clear days' notice of any planned changes in arrangements, and, in the event of sickness or other unplanned difficulty, to notify the relevant service immediately.

This contract will be reviewed with Mrs Mead, in the light of Margaret's changing needs, no later than 31 May 2001.

Signed: .... (for....agency/authority)

Contact address and phone number ....

Signed: .... (Mrs Ruth Mead)

Date ....

> In the event of any complaint about the services, please contact.......
> Mrs Mead has been provided with a copy of the Complaints Booklet.
> Independent advice can be sought from ...... Family Adviser with

[Organisation] at ....

The *support plan* would spell out in more detail such matters as:

- handover of medication
- clothing etc to be provided
- information exchange between services and mother
- emergency contact arrangements, including notification of and consultation about medical emergencies
- programme at the day centre
- programme at the respite unit.

An example of one area of the support plan is given in Box 9.7, which describes the respite care to be given to Margaret.

| Box 9.7 | **Programme at the respite unit** |

We are happy to welcome Margaret to our service. We will provide you with an information sheet about her activities and welfare when she leaves us at the end of each visit. We would appreciate an update about her health and recent activities when she comes to us; pro-formas have been provided.

Our aim is to make her stay enjoyable for Margaret and to allow you peace of mind while she is away from you. Please feel free to contact us at any time. You can of course visit if you wish to, but Margaret might get confused if you visit and leave without her, and I know you will have this in mind.

Activities vary with who is staying with us, and their health at the time, but we know that Margaret likes swimming, eating out and relaxing with music; she dislikes large crowds, loud noise and busy shops. We shall do our best to cater for her needs. We know that she likes to be up early, and to go to bed early, and we shall try to maintain the pattern she follows at home.

Should there be any incident, accident or health problem while she is with us, we will take any immediate action required, notify you as soon as possible and consult you about any further action required.

We are happy to discuss any issues or problems with you at a mutually convenient time.

Thank you for trusting Margaret to our care. She is a delightful young lady, and everybody here is very fond of her.

A personal profile details an individual's likes and dislikes and communication abilities. It would describe the person in all dimensions. Box 9.8 gives a personal profile for Margaret.

| Box 9.8 | **A personal profile plan** |

Margaret Mead: [Address, Date of Birth, Photo]
Clinical details: [medication, indications of prn medication, allergies, metabolic problems]
Margaret is a happy young lady who does not like to be fussed over but enjoys being with people—particularly one to one. She needs safe space to wander around but has to be watched when out of her chair because she is very unsteady. She greatly enjoys her food but is putting on weight: taste and variety need to be used to compensate for controlling quantity. She has no interest in television but does enjoy tuneful music—not too loud. She likes swimming, where one-to-one support is needed. She likes going out, particularly eating out, but becomes distressed in crowded places, especially crowded shops. She is upset by sudden noise.

When really contented, Margaret will chuckle uncontrollably for a few minutes. The immediate reason may be within Margaret as much as within her environment; but others can and do share her private pleasure. Although she is non-verbal and does not use signing, it is usually clear when she is hungry (burping noises or making for the kitchen) or thirsty (grabbing her empty drinking cup or someone else's). Pulling her bib up over her face is a good indication that she has had enough of an activity, or a person. When (if) she has had enough to eat, she will just turn her face away; but if she does this during the main course, do not assume she wants to miss the sweet course!

TERMINOLOGY AND CONTENT

The conventional term is 'care', and that term features prominently in both social and health services and in social security documents. There is much to be said for the alternative term 'support'. Support recognises that:

- many people with learning disabilities need prompting and encouragement rather than hands-on care
- there is a difference between doing to people what you have decided needs to be done, and supporting people in doing what they want to do
- when working with someone, there is an important job to be done in protecting and speaking up for their wider interests
- there should be a support network in which different people play different roles: from hands-on care to managing finances in a person's best interests.

Terminology has, as touched on earlier in this chapter, a wider impact in planning and monitoring services.

First, terminology can be used to base services in reality or it can be used to obscure the inability to deliver a service. If a hard-pressed service can really do not much more than keep people safe but bored, it helps nobody to say that 'our service seeks to empower clients by offering fulfilling choices'. Overstatement is irritating for clients, relatives and staff. This is not to decry the ambition to do better, but ambitions should start from reality.

Second, it matters greatly how service users are described. Even if diminishing terminology was not meant to damage, it can have that effect (Box 9.9).

Box 9.9	**The effect of diminishing terminology**

Arthur's personal hygiene was not always what it might have been. Staff described him as smelly when talking among themselves, then did so in the presence of other people's relatives and then told Arthur he was smelly. The few verbal clients picked up and used the same language. Eventually, Arthur was 'Smelly Arthur' to everyone and he began to play up to this weakness.

Meanwhile, nobody seriously addressed with Arthur how his personal hygiene could be improved. Once that point was reached, the risk was that Arthur would still keep his label, although the basis for the label had gone.

Third, the words used to describe a service and those who use the service can also mislead, to the disadvantage of both service and service users. If a service is described as catering for people with challenging behaviour, it will be assumed that this is the main presenting characteristic of those who live there or come there; others will then build their own picture of what challenging behaviour is. (Somebody who loses out on services through being very withdrawn will be labelled as very threatening—which is what challenging means to most people.) A rehabilitation unit will be assumed to provide a process of getting better for people who have in some ways got worse, and it may be associated with the popular notion of drying out after alcohol or substance abuse.

MONITORING   While choice has been a consistent theme in recent years, there is—apart from the old Scots choice of 'Will ye come in or will ye nae bother?'—precious little choice for most people for most of the time. The result has been a disinclination to monitor and a strong temptation to assume that all is well because all was well intended. For example, if the eventual out-of-county placement, found after searching for 6 months, might not be quite what had been intended, at least it is there, and it is not at all clear that there is anything else. If the private secure unit is a long way away and not the ideal long-term placement, it is a great deal more attractive than having someone back where nobody was willing to try even to contain him. A new unit would be far more expensive than simply filling the vacancy in that existing unit on the far side of the country. It is, therefore, worth asking why bother monitoring, rather than just waiting for the complaints and then trying again.

Theoretically, monitoring is essential. Practically, it might seem a luxury if there appears to be little than can be done to change things. There are a number of justifications for monitoring:

- If what is being paid for is not what is being achieved, the arrangements may not be cost effective even if they are cheap.
- A care assessment and plan can create an obligation to provide what has been stated to be needed; if it is not being provided, the law may be being broken.
- Unless provision is monitored, there is no way of knowing whether needs have changed or whether the service has changed while the needs have stayed the same. Monitoring detects if adjustments are required, even if they are not immediately possible
- Once the duty of care has been accepted, there is no legitimate escape from monitoring whether that duty of care is being discharged.
- A need for change does not necessarily mean a need for increased expenditure—some people will be found to need something different but not more expensive and even, perhaps, less expensive.

How and who of monitoring   There is an extensive literature defining quality, and an extensive literature about the means by which quality can be monitored; this chapter can only touch on some of the essentials. It is worth saying at the outset that in the context of person-centred planning, quality must be judged in relation to the person using the service. Margaret (Box 9.8) never looks at the television, and so ready access to multichannel TV is not a relevant quality measure for her. Unlike Charles, she hates shopping, so having visits to the local shops on her quality checklist misses the point. Were Charles or Margaret validly placed on the autistic spectrum, there would be question marks on the quality checklist against meeting lots of new people and doing lots of new things.

Essentially, effective monitoring requires the following:

- Staff know what is required of them, and what purpose is being served by their activities.
- Staff are trained to do what is required of them and in monitoring their own activity.
- Supervisors and managers know what is required of staff, and why, and focus on what is happening and what the results are.
- Any volunteers or other participants from outside the staff team are aware of the intended activities and the goals.
- Those who use the services are as far as possible themselves the custodians of their plans and are encouraged to give feedback on the fulfilment of the plans and the need to change the plans.
- Any involved relatives are also aware of intended activities and goals and are encouraged to comment—in the context of partnership in progress rather than just complaints when things go wrong.
- People who are relatively isolated are helped to acquire an independent advocate and preferably a circle of friends who share the plans and goals and are invited both to contribute and to comment.
- In the case of a residential service, neighbours who visit are given sufficient information about the service (rather than about individual people) to be able, and encouraged, to make suggestions.
- Staff, with outside involvement as required, have their own quality circle and work as a team (across shifts if there is a shift system) to monitor and improve quality.
- External auditors/inspectors/persons in control are briefed about the people, the plans, and the goals; they should have sufficient time to meet the people and spend time with them, as well as to check the environment and the paperwork.
- Use is made of the fresh insights that can be secured when there is a student or trainee present, and that person is invited to learn by challenging and not just learn by copying.
- Annual reviews are used to look at the lessons for the service, and not just the immediate circumstances of the service user.

- Where someone is using more than one service, or is living at home and using a service or services, service reviews and changes are shared with the other partners in support; the extent of support for the family is kept under review.
- Training needs are reviewed in line with service plans, and training for family carers is on offer—with shared training where appropriate. (For example, Mrs Mead was surprised to learn that the respite unit used oral diazepam where she was using rectal diazepam.)
- Senior managers do make use of incident reports, formal complaints, etc. as learning tools but also encourage and look at favourable comments and staff and visitor suggestions.
- Service users are encouraged to meet together to share insights and ideas, as well as being involved in staff selection and in formal monitoring arrangements.
- From time to time, senior managers share experience ('walking with'), in the family home, in a day service setting, in a respite unit or residential home, in a family placement, to see how it feels.

CONCLUSIONS Planning—even person-centred planning—needs to be kept in its place. Most people do not themselves choose to live completely according to plan and the few really determined self-planners can be quite odd. So forcing a rigid adherence to the plan can be counterproductive (Box 9.10). The opposite attitude was apparent in a psychiatric rehabilitation centre near Copenhagen. One of the clients was working at his bench with his dog lying beside him. When asked about this, the expected explanation might have been the centre's policy on pets or even a complete history of dog therapy. The Director was puzzled by the question. All she said was 'He is happier with the dog'. An outcome measure of happiness and a system with built-in flexibility cannot be bad.

Box 9.10	**A too rigid adherence to planning**

A special unit catered for young people who had experienced and caused major difficulties, and who hovered on the edge between the care system and the criminal justice system. The young people certainly had learning difficulties but only one, Jimmy, seemed to have a learning disability. After lunch, Jimmy picked up his book and started reading. The Director said, in a friendly but directive way, 'Jimmy, you are supposed to be outside now'. Jimmy, drawing attention to the obvious, replied 'I'm reading'. The Director, who was quite keen on his points system as a means of controlling behaviour, said firmly 'You will lose points'. Jimmy looked the Director in the eye and said, not unpleasantly, 'Stuff your points!'.

For the two case studies visited in this chapter, Charles and Margaret, a sensible shared system of person-centred planning and person-centred monitoring offers the framework for a happy life, but there has to be some spontaneity, some grasping of unexpected opportunities, some room to extend an experience that is obviously being enjoyed. Margaret has to be allowed to bring a tiring but enjoyable day to an early end in her comfortable and secure bed, even though another 2 hours of activity had been planned. Charles has to be allowed occasionally to stay up half the night because everything is much too interesting to abandon in favour of sleep.

The purpose of planning is to make happiness more likely. The purpose of monitoring is to check that those things are in place that are most likely to help achieve happiness, and that the person at the centre is indeed reasonably happy. However, it is the quality of the relationships, including the willingness to put the plan aside in the interests of the person's own judgement of happiness, which will deliver happiness, as a corollary of love even more than as a corollary of planning.

NOTE: This chapter was written some time before person-centred planning and other guidence was produced under the *Valuing people* implimentation programme.

REFERENCES

Deacon J 1977 Tongue tied. National Society for Mentally Handicapped Children, London

Department of Health 2001 Valuing people: a new strategy for learning disability for the 21st century (Cm 5086). The Stationery Office, London

Griffiths R 1988 Community care: agenda for action: a report to the Secretary of State for Social Services. HMSO, London

National Development Team 1988 The development of a contraction strategy for the Brockhall/Calderstones Unit in Lancashire. National Development Team

Spink K 1990 Jean Vanier and L'Arche: a communion of love. Darton, Longman and Todd, London

Wing L 1989 Hospital closure and the resettlement of residents: the case of Darenth Park Mental Handicap Hospital. Avebury Press, Aldershot

10 Older people with learning disabilities: moving on from institutional care

Anne Markwick and Alan Parrish

OVERVIEW
The commitment by the Government to raising standards and improving the quality of services for people with learning disabilities, leading to the White Paper *Valuing people* (Department of Health, 2001), was intended to enable people with learning disabilities to lead active and fulfilling lives in their communities and experience a range of activities, which includes leisure interests, friendships and other relationships. The intention is to provide good-quality services that promote independence, choice and inclusion and to allow a more meaningful life than that often achievable in an institutional setting.

This chapter discusses the effect these changes have had for older people with learning disabilities, who often have spent many years in an institutional setting. The problems and fears generated in this group by the proposed move from one environment to another are discussed, together with methods used to encourage them to make decisions for themselves. The chapter describes the issues that could arise from the time an institution has a date set for its closure until the time residents are resettled in more domestic style accommodation. The use of choice and personal autonomy to decline the new and opt for the old generates many questions; the response to these requires contributions from each and every member of a care team, and that all contributions should be valued and respected.

INTRODUCTION
Good-quality services must provide the right care for people with additional and complex needs. This includes people with severe and profound disabilities, people with a learning disability and epilepsy, those with learning disabilities and autism, people with challenging behaviour and older people with learning disabilities. This chapter concentrates on the last group and describes the movement from institutional care using the experiences of three people in this group. All three were over 70 years old and had collectively lived in institutional care in the north of England for over 120 years. The chapter describes the issues

that were addressed from the time that the institution they were living in had a date set for its closure until the residents were resettled in more domestic style accommodation.

The White Paper *Valuing people* (Department of Health, 2001) was the first legislation in the area of learning disability for 30 years, since the publication of the White Paper *Better services for the mentally handicapped* (Department of Health and Social Security, 1971). It has been warmly welcomed by just about everyone involved with this group, not only for its content but also for the attention that this paper gives to a group that is usually marginalised. *Valuing people* sets out how the Government will provide new opportunities for children and adults with learning disabilities and their families to live full and independent lives as part of their local communities.

There is no doubt that the pace of change involved in developing a new culture for the care of people with a learning disability has required a radical revision for many of personal attitudes and customs and managerial practices. The achievement of excellence in the design and delivery of services relies on the principle that both the service user and the service planner have mutual respect and understanding. This enables organisational barriers to be broken down and facilitates the forging of stronger links with all the services involved with the individual's care.

This chapter explains the story of the change and move from one environment to another and shows how the organisation involved was challenged in its own beliefs and values. The assumption is often that if the organisation believes it is offering people new opportunities and better ways of life involving choice and personal autonomy, the clients will see things the same way.

INSTITUTIONAL LIFE

For a person who has lived in an institution for much of their life, where systems and not individuals are the major factor of the service, it may not be easy to be confronted by a new way of life and suddenly find oneself having to make decisions and being asked for an opinion. The average person might find this easy to cope with, but for someone who has had greatly restricted choices for most of their life this can be very threatening. It is here that the education needs to start and this is a joint journey for both the service users and the carers.

This chapter is about the journey of three mature people, with a wealth of knowledge and a lifetime of experience of an institutional style of living, now being exposed to choice and autonomy. It is also about an organisation's journey from the institutional paradigm into valuing and respecting the individual, and the paradoxes that entailed. The complexity described above is illustrated using three people: Blanche Morris (Box 10.1), Bill Keen (Box 10.2) and Gladys Norwood (Box 10.3).

| Box 10.1 | **Blanche Morris** |

Blanche Morris was institutionalised at the age of 8 and her mother died 7 years later. Her estranged father was never a figure in her life and this resulted in her becoming devoted to her elder sister Pamela, who took over the parenting role during her early adulthood. Sadly, Pamela died 15 years prior to the closure of the institution and Blanche was forced to rely on the remaining siblings to whom she was never as close.

Her family were adamant that she should not be told about Pamela's death and insisted on sending Christmas and birthday cards in Pamela's name for all that time. Blanche could not read the cards for herself and would not have appreciated any handwriting changes, so the charade was easily played out. Blanche was told that her sister had become ill and was too poorly to visit. She accepted this but it seemed that she was then afraid that her sister might die and seemed to expect the news to come at any time. This was not an uncommon situation for people like Blanche. At the time the deception was started, staff would have felt under great pressure to cooperate with the family's wishes. As the years progressed the deception became more and more difficult to stop, especially as the family who kept regular contact with Blanche continued with it.

| Box 10.2 | **Bill Keen** |

Bill Keen was an only child and spent his early years at home with his family. He was institutionalised in his early twenties when his behaviour started causing concern. His parents were elderly by this time and although willing to continue caring for their son, they were physically unable to do so. His parents remained in close contact until they died and remained a big part of his life despite, in the latter years, seeing him infrequently through infirmity and the poor public transport to the isolated hospital.

He remained in the same hospital for the intervening 50 years, although he moved from ward to villa and back a number of times. During the moves, Bill maintained a strong friendship with two special friends, who remained close until they were resettled; this move prevented any regular contact other than an occasional phone call, which was restricted to when the staff were not already busy on the phone.

| Box 10.3 | **Gladys Norwood** |

Gladys Norwood was 23 years old when she was admitted to hospital and she remained there for the following 53 years. During that time her family were very conscientious and committed to maintaining their relationship with her. They visited regularly and often took her home for short periods. Her parents died in the mid-1980s and her brother and sister remained in close contact, visiting regularly and continuing to take her to their homes as often as was possible. Gladys had a particularly close bond with her brother Graham, who she looked to when making decisions for herself. He was a big influence on her and her instinct was always to defer to him in the first instance.

Gladys was a very quiet person who did not form close relationships with her peers, but she formed extremely close bonds with the less able residents and she was almost the sole carer for one young girl for many years. Molly, the young girl, was physically disabled and had a profound learning disability. Gladys carried out the main caring role for Molly and was devoted to her. Gladys restricted her own life in order to devote herself to her 'charge'. This relationship continued until Molly was moved to another hospital when her family relocated to the south of England. This had a devastating effect on Gladys in many ways. She became more introverted and for a period of about 6 months ate very little and lost a great deal of weight.

All three had been in institutional care for most of their lives. Collectively, this amassed to over 100 years.

The care that they experienced for the majority of those years had been traditionally institutional in that it centred around the organisation rather than the individuals who lived there. It was a segregated lifestyle that prevented and discouraged autonomy and choice and which served to disable rather than empower individuals. This commentary is not intended as a value judgement on those providing care at the time nor on those leading the overall organisation. Rather, it is intended to provide a backdrop to the lives of people who were institutionalised in previous generations, for whom life would certainly be very different today. Care at the time was given in a very different social, economic and political climate, and that must also be remembered when taking a look back. Indeed, there is no doubt that standards and attitudes have moved on enormously and that, latterly, people were becoming more familiar with the increased autonomy mentioned above, within some necessary practical constraints. It was not possible in a unit housing 20 people, for example, to ensure that all choices could be catered for every day.

However, as the resettlement programme progressed and the numbers of people living in each unit declined, staff were able to provide greater flexibility and choice for the remaining residents. In addition, staff generally were working within a different culture, where the prevailing attitude had shifted to respect for the residents and a genuine determination to improve everyday quality of life for everyone. In part, that is a contributory factor to the decision-making journey that these three people eventually took.

The White Paper *Better services for the mentally handicapped* was published in 1971. However, as is true for many policy documents, the changes were only felt in earnest some years after its publication. By the late 1980s, this fundamental shift in philosophy had meant that life was already changing for the better for many of the people living in hospital. This in itself, however, brought a new challenge to staff, who were faced with the need to examine, challenge and often change their own value systems. The staff team working with Bill, Blanche and Gladys were a very special group of people. They were very caring and sensitive and there is no doubt that they strove to improve the quality of the lives of the residents and that their commitment to them was enormous. The team was led by a very experienced nurse who was devoted to the ward and its residents and who created a very positive and homely environment. The team itself was not without its challenges, and they had had to face a new culture and new expectations of the service they provided. This was not always easy and they are to be commended for their commitment and energy to this end.

RESETTLEMENT   During this time, many people were moving to a 'better life' outside the institutions. However, some people experienced society's intolerance and hostility when they moved back into the community. This may have been caused by fear and ignorance, which was accentuated by the fact that for many years this group had been completely excluded from most communities. Consequently, there has been a steep learning curve for the general public and this has required a fundamental shift in attitude and values. Such changes in attitude take time to make an impact but, in the main, many people with learning difficulties now lead full and rewarding lives. This is in stark contrast with those who do remain on the margins of our society, suffering prejudice, bullying, insensitivity and discrimination, whether within an institution or in a community.

The resettlement process, as it was known, which moved people from institutions to a more ordinary lifestyle, did not allow people to have complete freedom or control over their own destiny, and many found themselves moving into groups chosen for them and away from the friendships which they had built up over the years. The latest White Paper *Valuing people* (Department of Health, 2001) updates the Government's commitment to people with learning disabilities. It shows how they will meet this commitment by ensuring that local councils, the National Health Service (NHS), voluntary organisations and, most importantly, people with learning disabilities and their families, work closely together to provide new opportunities for those with learning disabilities to lead full and active lives. It is intended that this group should be given more control over their own destiny, which they have been denied in past decades.

Plans to close the hospital that was home to Bill, Blanche and Gladys for so many years were part of the strategic approach that was being implemented across the country. A date was set by the management team, in line with the predicted date of completion of the resettlement process. Large numbers of people from the hospital had already been successfully resettled and the staff had learned a great deal about how to involve people as far as possible in the decision making and to give people the autonomy that was their right. Every effort was made to make this process as positive as possible for the people who were being resettled. Protracted periods of familiarisation were built in and both the old and new staff teams were encouraged to work in both the hospital and the new homes to facilitate the development of new relationships and to build the confidence of the people who were moving. As the numbers of remaining residents reduced, the staff who remained in the hospital were able to work in new ways, often giving people more freedom and choice than had previously been possible as a result of lower staff to resident ratios and greater numbers of people in each area generally. This meant that staff needed new skills and appropriate attitudes, and the support that these required. The staff team described above enjoyed this new way of working, and it is possible that this contributed to the difficulty they later experienced in coming to terms with their own losses.

Resistance to resettlement

New homes were identified as suitable for Bill, Blanche and Gladys. All three and the families of Blanche and Gladys were involved in assessing the suitability and desirability of the homes through visits and contact with the new staff teams. At first the families did not want their relatives to move from the security, as they saw it, of the hospital. The resistance that was initially experienced was not uncommon amongst families and was born out of fear of change and the unknown, some fear about society's reaction to people who are perceived as different, and some disbelief that, after all these years, the hospital really would close. It must have felt, particularly after institutional life had changed so much for the better in the recent past, as if the authorities were determined to fix something that appeared, in their eyes, not to be broken. Staff spent considerable time discussing with the families the new philosophy and the benefits for the individuals of the move into more ordinary housing. Commonly, the experience after the moves was that families felt very strongly that the new way of life was better and that, with hindsight, they would not choose to return to 'the old days'. However, many described the painful process that the change had been, which is something that we all face during periods of change and uncertainty.

When a date for hospital closure was set, this became a target for completion of the resettlement and seemed to be the point at which the relatives realised that closure was indeed going to happen. Reactions of the families and the individuals varied (Boxes 10.4–10.6).

Box 10.4	**Blanche Morris: refusal of resettlement**

Blanche's family soon became enthusiastic supporters of the move; although they did not live close enough to be frequent visitors, they took part in the process as far as was possible. Blanche herself frequently spoke of her fear that she was to be moved to the local cottage hospital, where she was afraid people only went to die. Staff's reassurance did not entirely stop the fear and even frequent visits to her new home did not fully persuade her that this would not happen until soon before the day she finally moved for good.

Box 10.5	**Bill Keen: refusal of resettlement**

Bill had no family to support him through these major life changes and he had refused to speak to the advocates who offered to work on his behalf. He remained clear throughout the process that he was happy within the hospital and there he wished to stay. He was happy to go and visit the proposed new home and enjoyed the novelty and meeting new people but stated clearly that he did not want to leave the staff team he felt very fond of or the friendships he had had for so many years.

Box 10.6	**Gladys Norwood: refusal of resettlement**

Gladys's family gradually became more used to the idea of her moving and visited the new home again. They became more supportive and actively encouraged the move. Unfortunately, Gladys held on to her belief that her brother wanted her to stay and this she referred to in support of her continued resistance to the move. She consistently reported that whilst the new home was very nice she didn't want to live there—'it wasn't her home'.

Response to a refusal of relocation

What happened between the refusal to move and the subsequent successful relocation of all three of these remarkable people was complex and interesting and challenged the very value base of the organisation. In describing the process in this way, there is a danger that it becomes oversimplified and that the complexity is not appreciated. A number of significant things happened almost concurrently and this is impossible to describe faithfully on paper. It is also difficult to describe fully the time, effort and commitment given, particularly by the front-line staff. There was a very fine balance between giving people the appropriate information with which to make a very difficult decision and bullying and cajoling people into doing what was considered to be 'right'.

At a fairly early stage in the resettlement process, it became very clear to the organisation that these three people were giving a straightforward message. These new homes were all right to visit but they would prefer to stay in the hospital and were quite content to continue living there. It was the home they knew and in which they were happy and they preferred it 'warts and all'. Despite all the efforts at persuasion and imparting copious amounts of information to enable an informed decision, they independently stuck to their position. The attempts at persuasion were based on a firm belief on the part of the staff that the new way of life offered to them would ultimately be preferable and beneficial. It was in no way an exercise in power and control or the wish for an expedient or economically preferable outcome. However, regardless of the staff's motivation, they stood firm. They continued to visit their prospective new homes but remained adamant that the visits were to be just that. They were given absolute control over whether they continued to visit, how long the visits lasted and when they returned home.

During this time, a discussion took place in the senior management team of the organisation that centred around what to do about the three euphemistically termed 'reluctant movers'. It had become painfully clear that these people were more than reluctant and had simply refused to consider moving. That faced the team with the startling revelation that a challenge was being mounted to the very value base of the organisation. The question was whether the organisation truly valued and respected people with a learning disability, as it purported to do, or whether this only applied while people were making judgements that fell into line with the organisation's own collective opinion. Could it face the issue and consider what the alternatives were or would it default to the paternalistic perspective where 'we know best'? This provoked a heated debate, and the outcome was that the team was prepared to respect the wishes of the three and, while they were unable to promise them a lifetime remaining on the ward where they currently lived, a commitment was made to provide for them on site if they insisted that this was what they wanted. An ensuing flow of activity looked into the implications of this decision and how to underpin a philosophical commitment with the physical ability to deliver the promises.

At a similar time, the Chief Executive went to visit Blanche, Bill and Gladys to ascertain for himself their level of appreciation of the situation and to evaluate the current position. The visit was an interesting example of someone with sophisticated verbal skills being entirely disabled by three people who managed to use their whole selves to communicate their very clear message. They chose to alternate between standing by their stance and gently but firmly distracting the Chief Executive with interjections of their own interests or special belongings. Blanche took him to her room and showed him her most precious belongings. Bill kept leaving the room to ensure that the whole staff team were aware that he was having a chat with who he referred to as 'the boss man'. Blanche sat quietly with her eyes down. She answered politely all the questions she was asked. Almost every answer, however, was 'Thank you but I like it here'. They expertly distracted the

Chief Executive's ability to delve into this issue and politely but firmly showed him his own deficits in terms of real communication.

Virtually concurrently with this, it was felt by the multiprofessional care team to be appropriate to break the news to Blanche of her sister's death. She had recently started to ask openly if she was dead, and the staff felt increasingly uncomfortable perpetuating the lie. The family remained unable to accept this but it was felt to be important enough to go against the wishes of the family in a genuine attempt to benefit Blanche in the longer term. This decision was not taken lightly and a great deal of preparation took place before the news was broken. A bereavement counsellor became involved with Blanche and the staff team all agreed to take part in a bereavement workshop, which was seen to be a crucial part of the preparation. The workshop turned out to be a revelation to everyone and resulted in a significant number of staff recognising, for the first time, that the closure of the hospital was almost as big an event for them as it was for the residents. It transpired that the staff had been harbouring the same secret belief that somehow the hospital would not really close, that something somehow would halt it just at the last minute. This clearly mirrored the relatives' and the residents' beliefs that had been demonstrated in the preceding weeks. The closure was to mark the end of a significant part of everyone's life and this was the realisation that whatever the future held there was no holding on to the past. This was a pivotal moment. The staff team were incredibly brave, open and honest during this and the subsequent period and it is to their credit that they were able to come to terms with their own loss and to work through it in order to support the users of their services.

In the event it seemed that somehow Blanche had suspected the truth and it appeared to be almost a relief to her that she would no longer be constantly expecting the bad news. Perhaps in some way Blanche had feared that she would not be there for Pamela if she moved and then Pamela suddenly recovered and came back. She was, of course, upset by the news, and the staff and the counsellor played a central role in supporting her through the difficult time. She chose to have a private memorial service to remember Pamela and she chose a brightly coloured ribbon, which she wore in memory of her sister. Blanche remained dignified throughout the process. The people who supported her are to be commended for their sensitivity of approach and their detailed preparation and planning.

Successful relocation No trumpets or fanfares marked these pivotal moments in the process of closing the hospital. Its activities largely continued in a very similar way. The visits to their prospective homes continued for Blanche, Bill and Gladys, and the work with the families continued in the same pattern.

However, something seemed to have fundamentally shifted. There was an overt commitment to the valuing of all three people that had previously been hidden or assumed. Following the shakiness that accompanied the difficult organisational dilemma of paternalism versus autonomy, the Trust reached a new level of confidence in its values and beliefs, which was, in a way, freeing. The residents were still in control of the process of visits to their prospective new homes and the efforts to provide them with the right information to make their decisions continued. The approach continued with small steps, calculated risks and fall back positions. This was underpinned by the demonstration to the residents that the staff and the organisation would be true to their word and the control was, finally, truly with them.

The results were quite remarkable. Within 3 weeks, Bill had agreed to move to his new home for a trial period of 3 months and he has remained there happily ever since. He maintains intermittent contact with his old friends and has made more friends in the local village through his day activities and the clubs that he attends. Blanche moved within a similar period, having established that she genuinely would not be going to the cottage hospital to die, that she could take her possessions with her and that her family would continue to be a part of her life. She is settled and happy and has forged strong relations with the new staff team.

Gladys continued to visit the new house and opted very soon to stay overnight. She suffered a period of serious ill-health, which it was feared would jeopardise or at least hold up the process. However, she gently but firmly let it be known that she did not want to stop the visits and so they continued with the necessary additional support built in. Her family began to visit her there and she began bringing items of her own to leave in her new room. She began to refer to her 'new room' when back in the hospital. One night, some weeks later, she asked the staff in the new home to bring the remaining belongings she had and she has remained there ever since.

CONCLUSIONS Looking back over the story of resettlement given here, it is fascinating that it took a firm, overt commitment from the organisation to allow the decision to be truly in the hands of the residents, for them to be able to make the decision that the organisation had been trying, seemingly too hard, to enable them to make in the first place. Several other factors were important in the change. The importance of the family relationships cannot be discounted. However, it was also important for the people immediately involved to be given access to information about their lives, even if that could be painful, in order that they could be fully in charge of their own decisions. The decision of Blanche's family, with the kindest of motives, to protect her by withholding information was based on the paternalistic frame that it was vital to move beyond. It must be recognised that sometimes actions taken to protect us can disable us in the process.

At the time of the resettlement issue, the organisation management felt that it had learned a lot about enabling people to move and had a high level of expertise in that process. It is ironic that it was only by coming to terms with the wishes of the three residents and allowing their true enablement and empowerment that the most fundamental aspect of moving on became clear. The journey the organisation took was nothing compared with the journey that Blanche, Bill and Gladys took, but each journey was dependent upon the other. What is certain is that the organisational journey will leave an important legacy that will benefit many people in the future, and that the personal journeys taken by the three remarkable people have taken them and their families to happy and fulfilled lives.

REFERENCES Department of Health 2001 Valuing people: a new strategy for learning disability for the 21st century (Cm 5086). The Stationery Office, London

Department of Health and Social Security 1971 Better services for the mentally handicapped (Cmnd 4683). HMSO, London

11 Changing philosophy in learning disability

Brian Kay

OVERVIEW This chapter considers the change in the philosophical background of provision for people with learning disabilities particularly in the 20th century. Changes over time in the theoretical basis of care for those with learning disabilities are discussed, including the move from a duty/ethics basis to a rights-based philosophy. The effect of changing attitudes in society in general is examined in terms of changes in government policy and legislation, the implementation of those changes and the effect these have had on both the service providers and the service users.

INTRODUCTION There are two main threads that have been apparent throughout this book. First is the theme of constant change, and second is the development over time of thought and the way in which the nature of learning disability has been understood and presented. Much of this change is mirrored in the language that has been used, from terms like idiot, imbecile, feebleminded through mental subnormality, mental handicap and to the current usage of learning difficulties or learning disabilities. People with learning disabilities have been called patients, inmates, trainees, residents, clients and, more recently, 'service users'. Chapter 7 gave a detailed account of how services have developed, in line with the concurrent legislation and government papers and reflects how this might have directed the approach to care for a typical service user over the years.

MODELS FOR UNDERSTANDING LEARNING DISABILITY How we approach people with learning disability is largely dependent upon how we see them, how we understand the nature of their needs and the context in which we frame our responses. During the 20th century, there have been four main models or paradigms for understanding learning disability (Kay, 1994).

The medical model

From the early 1900s until the 1950s, the model was primarily the medical model, which was essentially a custodial model. Learning disability was seen as a 'disease' or medical condition. This view was enhanced where diagnosis could be made by identified medical syndromes such as Down syndrome or phenylketonuria. Those individuals who came into contact with statutory agencies often found themselves placed in institutions (hospitals) under the care of doctors and asylum attendants (later nurses). Apart from a small number of conditions such as phenylketonuria or congenital hypothyroidism, where there was recognised medical treatment, people were cared for but there was no concept of treatment. It was not until the mid-1950s, when medical treatment and advances in mental health care started to highlight the lack of medical intervention in learning disabilities, that the medical model was seriously questioned. As mental health care moved forward, learning disability became a less rewarding field for the medical profession.

The behavioural model

At this point, an alternative model was needed. If learning disability was not a disease or a medical condition, or was not amenable to medical treatment, then what was it? How do we understand it? It was at about this time that the work of behavioural psychologists such as B F Skinner was coming to the fore (Skinner, 1953). Behavioural psychologists, initially in the USA, developed techniques for replacing inappropriate behaviours or behavioural patterns with more appropriate and acceptable ones. These approaches, initially developed on animals, were adapted to use with people, and individuals with learning disabilities were among the first groups to benefit from this. (The more cynical may also note the need around this time for psychologists to develop a professional role and identity.) The move from an endless round of conducting intelligence quotient (IQ) tests to actually leading successful therapeutic interventions was a welcome and positive development for clinical psychologists in learning disabilities. For the first time, there was a professional group offering tangible advice and support to people with learning disabilities and their carers. Behavioural approaches became major news. However, there were two major drawbacks to this approach. First, the emphasis on inappropriate behaviours tended, inevitably, to focus on negative actions. Inappropriate behaviours, aggression, violence, self-injury, damage to property, screaming, 'smearing' and overt sexual behaviour started to become the way in which people with learning disabilities were perceived—the focus was on 'problem' behaviours, which soon, with the softening of language, became behaviours that challenge or 'challenging behaviours'. Second, while this model seemed more applicable than the medical model, it was, in the long term, equally inaccurate. For a significant percentage of people with learning disabilities, there was no presentation of challenging behaviours; they were quiet, meek and gentle and many had very profound physical disabilities and needed no 'behavioural' intervention.

The social model   Very often the features that brought people with learning disabilities to the attention of agencies was their lack of social skills. Their need for support and assistance with personal hygiene, eating and dressing was what placed the demand upon support and care services. This awareness of their needs was paralleled by developments in society, which in the mid-1970s was focussed much more on individual freedom, expression and the development of rights. The inception of social services departments and social workers in the 1970s added to the development of the third model, the social model. In this context, many challenges were seen as 'social handicaps' and people with learning disabilities were seen as socially handicapped or socially inadequate; thus, terminology moved from medical terminology, such as idiot, imbecile, feeble-minded or moral defective, through the more psychologically led terms such as mental subnormality (based primarily on IQ) and on to the concept of mental handicap. Again there were parallel developments in professional roles and functions—the move from the medical model had also meant that people were starting to question the role of learning disability (mental handicap) nurses. The Jay Report in 1979 (Department of Health, 1979) identified that (residential) social work may be the more appropriate base upon which to provide support and services.

This was in line with other social and political developments, as described in Chapter 7. The growth of normalisation and social role valorisation emphasised the importance of growth and development occurring in the home in small, family units and this led directly to the move from large institutional settings for people with learning disabilities. The basis of the behavioural approach gradually shifted from behaviour 'modification' to utilising behavioural theory to underpin learning and teaching, with the emphasis upon social skill development. This process led to a model of working *with* people with learning disabilities rather than 'operating' upon them. The somewhat harsh approach of behaviour modification became more a form of 'gentle teaching'. Again, for the more cynical, this development was in parallel with the development of social work as a profession and the shift in learning disability nursing, which was enshrined in the 1982 Registered Nurse of the Mentally Handicapped syllabus (National Boards for England and Wales, 1982).

These changes must also be seen in parallel with societal developments, the social revolution of the 1960s and 1970s, with the striving for a more equitable society (often described as the rise of the meritocracy) and the major changes in legislation with laws relating to racial discrimination, sexual discrimination, divorce, abortion, sexual preferences and practices and suicide. These all pointed towards an approach based more on 'rights' in the way in which society was structured. In addition, lower unemployment and a more affluent society supported a trend towards a more charitable view of disadvantaged or vulnerable people, which made the concept of 'social handicap' more acceptable.

The educational model

Thus, the scene was set for the fourth model for understanding learning disability, the educational model. This logically grew out of both the behavioural and the social models. The former was based on the rationale that people with learning disability behaved inappropriately and exhibited challenging behaviours because they had learned to behave in this way: if these are learned behaviours, it is, therefore, the learning process that has been dysfunctional and needs remedying or educating. Similarly, the social model said people with learning disabilities lacked the appropriate social skills because they had difficulty in learning, therefore, have special educational needs.

Much of this was sustained by the Warnock Report (Committee of Enquiry, 1978), which identified 'special educational need' and recommended far-reaching changes in educational policy and legislation, including a huge increase in special educational provision, extension of school ages and much greater integration in education. Again we should not perhaps overlook the fact that in this period there were falling rolls, that a significant number of teacher training colleges closed and that the teaching profession was significantly under threat. Consequently, a report advocating the need to increase the number of teachers and fundamentally alter the role of teaching (from the 'three Rs' to 'preparing people for life') was not entirely untimely from an educationalist and teaching viewpoint.

The current position

As we might expect, none of the four models were entirely satisfactory or self-sufficient. However, they did offer a way of viewing and understanding the nature of learning disability and the people who were thus labelled and, most importantly, they were congruous with the changes in view and structure that were occurring in Western and most specifically in British society.

Many people are not excited by this type of historical and sociological analysis and approach to learning disability. However, it is valuable both in order to understand from where the current views and approach have developed and to explain why further developments are likely to be of a certain form over the next 10 years. As we have seen from the preceding chapters, the philosophy and the approach to supporting people with learning disabilities are in the process of fundamental and radical change, not only pragmatically but also in terms of the paradigm that underpins how services may develop. In order to understand this and to develop with it, it is valid to look at the nature of the change and the context in which it is occurring.

SHIFT IN POWER   One of the most significant flaws in or disadvantages to the four models is that they are clearly 'professions' based. They are overtly paternalistic and assume that it should be professionals or agencies that define the nature of the people they work with and the way in which services are provided. Whether it be psychiatrists, doctors, nurses, social workers or teachers, it is clear that they have vested interests and it is apparent from our exploration of the models that there may well be external agendas for professionals, which relate to the status and development of the professions, that influence this process. It may inevitably be the case that where the professionals are defining both the nature of learning disability and the form and structure of service provision, this may well be some distance from the experiences, understanding, needs and aspirations of the people with learning disability themselves.

In real terms what we are examining is a power base. The models are clearly based on a paradigm where the basis of power and control rests with the professionals and the service providers. The fundamental and radical shift is the movement of that power base from professionals and providers to where it should be—with the individuals themselves. As considered a number of times in the preceding chapters, the fundamental basis of person-centred planning is that control and design of support provision rests with the person with a learning disability and their chosen circle of support. The challenge is to facilitate this and sustain its evolution into common practice throughout society—no mean feat!

No mean feat because the challenge is both complex and immensely difficult. As discussed in Chapter 9, on planning and monitoring of care, this challenge is far more than paying lip service to a few simple words and ideas and requires much more than introducing a few new forms and developing some new jargon. For most involved in this area, it involves a sea change in total outlook and approach.

Of course, the biggest challenge of all is actually identifying exactly what the aspirations, wants and needs are of those people who invite the professionals to participate in their support.

So where do the models leave us? We have not quite spanned the gap between the professions-based models and the person-centred approach. There are two main factors that have evolved since the 1960s that will assist this move: the shift from a deontological paradigm to rights-based philosophy and the change in our understanding of disability itself.

The shift from duty/ethics to a rights-based philosophy

Part of the ethos of most professions is some element of 'calling' or vocational basis, which is heavily intertwined with concepts around duty and obligation. The concept of a duty of care, for example, has perplexed many professionals in their practice and has often been used as a rationale for some highly paternalistic and even restrictive interventions that have frequently not matched, in any way, the wishes of the individual. We see this highlighted on a number of occasions in Chapter 5.

The deontological paradigm relies heavily on concepts of duty and is underpinned by many tenets found in most of the world religions and philosophies: a duty of care for fellow beings and for life in general. There is an element of self-sacrifice and a view that every individual should to some extent forego their own wishes and desires for the benefit of others.

At the other end of the continuum is an extreme view of rights: people have a right to freedom, to self-expression and to happiness. At its most extreme, this can be a philosophy of hedonism and selfishness, but most people fall somewhere along the middle of this continuum. Certainly, changes in society in the UK in the 1960s and 1970s saw an enormous growth in the acceptance of a more rights-based philosophy and rationale. The position on this continuum where individuals stand is often related to the generation in which they grew up. This is often seen in seminar groups covering three generations and it can usually be related to our own experiences within the family. The change in position can be demonstrated by asking a group of mixed generations one simple question. 'One or both of your elderly parents are no longer able to care for themselves properly and are at risk; they can no longer live alone. What should happen? Who should care for them?'

For those reared before World War II, there is no difficulty here. Brought up on a deontological philosophy they will see it as their duty to care for their parents. They will adapt their home to take them in and care for them and they will, in the main, do this willingly and happily (a chance to repay the debt they owe for their own care and protection as children). It would be viewed as a matter of duty. Children reared in the 1970s and 1980s have no such pressure of obligation: 'You will have to go in to a home. We will pick a satisfactory one with a good standard of care; we will visit you regularly and check that you are being properly looked after'. These children were brought up in an era based far more on rights than on duty. They have a right to their own independence, their own life and should not have to be burdened by their parents. The parents cannot complain about this; they reared them and are responsible for the development of their philosophy on life. Many of those brought up in the 1950s and 1960s would agree with them anyway, believing that each person is responsible for their own care and needs and should not wish to impose upon their off-spring: after all they have their own families and their own responsibilities. However, this generation is also more likely to feel a sense of duty and obligation to care for their parents, but not as willingly as the previous generation. In fact, they might meet their obligations and fulfil their duty, but not without some resentment and some sense of sacrifice and inconvenience. What about my rights?

Obviously, this is a sweeping generalisation, and different families may well have different responses in any generation, but it does illustrate the shift in perspective that has occurred.

Clearly what is seen is a continuum and not two separate ideologies. Many rights-based protagonists understand and expound the importance of obligations and of responsibility to others, and likewise many deontologists recognise the need for individual identity and expression. Nevertheless, most people can identify where they stand on this continuum.

Duty and rights in the development of community care

In fact, the process of evolution from deontology to rights and the confusion that can result can be seen quite starkly in the development of community care. Many people have found the legislation and subsequent outcomes quite perplexing, but from inception to implementation 'community care' is almost exactly coterminous with the period when the shift between ideologies was evolving.

It is often extremely useful to identify where people do stand on this when discussing service provision or planning care. Unless the basic premise that people are working from is established, conflict and confusion can ensue. For example, in the early days of the movement towards community care, new and enthusiastic staff who were involved in consultation exercises, or debates with local communities where group homes were being planned, would expound the rights-based philosophy: people with learning disabilities have the right to the same services and lifestyle as any other member of the community. They would be somewhat nonplussed when local citizens asked 'Says who?' or even more directly 'No they don't'. Many such reluctant citizens would argue a deontological viewpoint: 'Such people need care and we meet our duty to provide that—we pay the taxes and rates that provide hospitals and pay staff wages'. Though here of course the staff were implying that the community had a 'duty' to respond to these 'rights'.

Community care in Britain was planned and envisioned under the Government of Margaret Thatcher. Mrs Thatcher was a strong deontologist who made little attempt to conceal her view that the national philosophy had gone awry in the 1960s—too much emphasis on rights had created a 'dependent' culture where people expected the State to provide everything. In this view, people were abdicating their responsibility for and duty to their family and their fellow human beings to the State. They had a right to work and, therefore, a right to child care; they had a right to freedom and, therefore, obligations to their family should be met through state support and provision. The Community Care Act was conceived with a view to redressing this balance. The State should support people to meet their own obligations: there would be help to modify homes so that people could care for their own ailing or dependent relatives and so forth. If the individual did not wish to meet their own 'obligations', then the State would be willing to do it for them but they would have to pay for it. The State would provide homes, services, etc., but there would be a charge. People who had assets would have to convert them to pay for service provision. These were some of the premises that underpinned the inception of this Act. So, where does the confusion come in? Basically, because although the Act was envisioned and developed under Margaret Thatcher, it was implemented under John Major. Major was a different generation; as a product more of the 1950s and 1960s, he was a firm believer in a much more rights-based approach (a 'classless society'). The weakness in the rights-based philosophy in the UK had always been its lack of a credible provenance. The deontologists have a huge spectrum of established material to call on to justify their legitimacy: the Bible, the Koran, the Talmud, etc. There was a plethora of documents established over many centuries identifying a person's duty to their fellow beings and in fact to all sentient beings: our duty of care and of responsibility to others.

In the UK, in the absence of a Bill of Rights, the only basis ordinarily available is common law, most of which traditionally is based upon precedent. Major recognised this early on and endeavoured to legislate for this with the development of charters such as the Citizens' Charter and the Patients' Charter. If they became accepted and utilised within society, they would have gradually become the basis for a rights-based approach. The implementation of the Community Care Act by Major's Government was far more user friendly and rights orientated than had been originally intended by its founders; sadly, it was never funded on the basis of the volume of usage it would facilitate if viewed from a rights perspective.

People did have the right not to be incarcerated in large institutions, whether they be psychiatric hospitals or mental handicap hospitals. However, closing hospitals without making alternative provisions for vulnerable members of society is not without its problems.

The development of rights-based approaches, in general, coincided with or even facilitated the development in our understanding of and approach to learning disability. The concepts of normalisation (Wolfensberger, 1972) and, later, social role valorisation are very much based on the rights and entitlements of the individual. As with any other development of ideas, there were those who became fanatical and extremist in their views and actions, and some aspects of normalisation became corrupted, or at least misdirected, by a less-considered more obdurate fixation on its tenets. All types of anomaly were perpetrated in the name of normalisation. At the extreme, for example, in the USA, was the demand for the right to be executed for learning disabled people who found themselves on 'death row', having been 'normalised' through the legal process. Even in the UK in the late 1980s, when concern was expressed about the increasing number of people with learning disabilities finding their way into the criminal and penal system, one rationale was normalisation: it is 'normal' for people who offend to go to prison, irrespective of their level of intellect or cognition. To some extent, such extreme interpretations of normalisation started to bring the fundamental logic and correctness of this approach into disrepute.

Understanding disability

The second fundamental development in thought that gave rise to the shift from professions-based to person-centred approaches is in our understanding of disability.

The shift in approach to and understanding of disability can be traced back to its origins in the 1970s, although it was in the 1990s that the real impact was felt. It was this key factor, perhaps more than anything else, that revolutionised not only the current approach to learning disabilities but also, more broadly, the approach to all aspects of service development and provision. When this approach was first expounded, its proponents were seen almost as heretics, trying to undermine the development of normalisation. The problem with normalisation had always been interpretation. For some it meant to treat people who had specific challenges or needs as if they were normal (i.e. just like we would treat anyone else), which might mean ignoring their special needs or challenges. For others, it meant to try and 'make' people normal—to force them somehow to behave as everyone else did. Even Wolfensberger himself had intimated that the ultimate measure of success of normalisation in human services would be realised when we did not need any special services for groups of individuals in society (Wolfensberger, 1972). The downside of all this was, in essence, to create the opposite of what was intended: actually to deny a person's individuality or identity.

The more there is a campaign on behalf of people with a disability, the more society 'normalises' them, the more patronising it becomes. If a person has a challenge or specific need, that need is part of their identity, part of who they are, and they do not necessarily want to have that part of their identity ignored or denied. In a sense, what developed was the growth of a rights-based philosophy: a person has a right to their disability and to have it recognised. Perhaps the most cogent demonstration of this was the debate that grew around the surgical application of cochlear implants. Many people who had grown up entirely with deafness had become part of their deaf community—they could communicate using sign language and they could attend social, recreational and employment activities for the deaf. They were in the main, by their own estimation, not disabled; they lived a normal life within their own chosen communities. The cochlear implant would, of course, enable them to hear to some extent—it would make them 'normal' in the context of a hearing society—but many rejected this as they did not have any sense of being 'abnormal' or 'incomplete'. Within the context of their society, they were normal and they had a right to be themselves. This is an amazingly powerful rationale and argument, which shocked and challenged many peoples' view and understanding both of disability and of the real meaning of rights. Although there are many other examples, the cochlear implant debate is the most profound and the most telling.

THE CURRENT ETHOS

It is from this kind of debate and this revolution of ideas that the current basis has been reached, from which our understanding and approach to service development and provision must proceed. If nothing else, it highlights that it is not for the professional to legislate service provision. Professionals have to listen to the people, who may or may not choose to use services, to define how those services should develop and function.

This situation is not even that radical for the deontologists. If the underpinning rationale of deontology is service to others or obligation, then what is wrong with the recipients of services defining what service is needed, how it should be provided and in what context and on what terms? It is entirely logical.

Of course there is still the enormous challenge, regardless of philosophical stance, of enabling communication. How does the person with a learning disability communicate their wishes, aspirations and needs? How does the provider or respondent learn to communicate or to identify what he or she is being asked to offer? Services based entirely on models, paradigms or high-flying esoteric principles have every likelihood of going seriously astray, in spite of good intentions.

Chapter 9 makes this point most effectively: there has to be some pragmatism and some recognition of practicalities. In fact, where there is imperfection, as there always must be, it will be in the service provider, who is 'disabled' in their ability to communicate with and reach their service user, rather than in the individual seeking the support of the service.

Before leaving this discussion altogether, it is interesting to reflect upon the difficulties this whole process has created for everyone involved. The dilemmas faced by the 'professionals'—doctors, nurses, social workers and therapists—have been highlighted; many have worked lengthy careers in the field of learning disabilities and feel they have campaigned fervently on behalf of people with learning disabilities. In spite of living through this period of change, many find some challenges in coming to terms with the inevitable outcomes of this evolution. Perhaps one of the major developmental points on this journey has been the establishment of 'supported living' models. It has been most gratifying after so many years to see people with learning disabilities living as tenants in their own homes, and even owning their own homes, but it has also been fascinating to see how much difficulty some professionals have had in grasping this development.

For some professionals it has been difficult to accept that they do not have right of entry but should be invited in. Others do not understand why support providers cannot prevent people from accessing their own kitchen (on the grounds of safety) or that support providers cannot arbitrarily move people from one house or service to another on the basis of perceived need.

If this process has created challenges for professionals, it has done no less for parents, relatives and carers. In some ways, the evolution has been positive, and relatives and carers have found themselves more likely to be consulted and involved. Professionals have been less inclined to see their roles as protecting individuals from their relatives and more inclined to consult and to listen. In the main (with the possible exception of debates around 'village communities'), professionals and statutory agencies have recognised the need to work in partnership with relatives and carers. Certainly in recent years, governments have been more inclined to consult relatives of people with learning disabilities (sometimes to the chagrin of some people with learning disabilities, who have felt, much like other increasingly independent individuals, that their relatives and carers do not necessarily reflect their own wishes and aspirations).

Finally, of course, this evolution has presented major challenges for people with learning disabilities themselves, who suddenly find themselves being consulted or asked to make choices for the first time, with little explanation or opportunity to develop the prerequisite skills or necessary support networks.

This, then, is the point reached now in the development of ideas and philosophy. It is encapsulated in the White Paper *Valuing people* (Department of Health, 2001). Developments over the next decades from this basis and through the various implementation guidelines and task forces will shape service provision to provide support and care for people with learning disabilities into the foreseeable future. The basic structure to underpin this will be the person-centred planning approach, of which the most comprehensive exposition is found in Sanderson et al. (2000).

CONCLUSIONS

This chapter has covered the development of ideas in learning disability in some considerable length because I feel strongly that it is important to understand how such developments come about. Some comments have been overtly political at times, unapologetically because the provision of services is a political issue. Some aspects described may be seen to be speculative and open to interpretation; this is fine, I do not claim infallibility. The main desire has been to generate some thought and consideration of how we have arrived at the current stage in our journey. The consideration of why learning disability is perceived in its current form is not simply pragmatic in terms of provision of services; in fact, in some ways that is the least important aspect of it. Obviously, receiving support and services is paramount to individuals trying to make their way in society today. A roof over our heads, food in our stomachs and some sense of self-esteem and value are important, as is some degree of economic security, but, arguably, the old institutions provided most of that. The changes that have occurred and are occurring are much more than that, which the chapters in this book have illustrated only too well.

REFERENCES

Committee of Enquiry 1978 Special educational needs (Cmd 7212) (The Warnock Report). HMSO, London

Department of Health 1979 Jay Report: Committee of Enquiry into Mental Handicap Nursing and Care (Cmd 74680). HMSO, London

Department of Health 2001 Valuing people: a new strategy for learning disability for the 21st century (Cm 5086). The Stationery Office, London

Kay B 1994 Helping individuals with mental handicap or emotional dependence In: Webb P (ed) Health promotion and patient education: a professional's guide. Chapman & Hall, London, pp 272–292

National Boards for England and Wales 1982 Syllabus of training. Professional register Part 5: registered nurse of the mentally handicapped. Bocardo Press, Oxford

Sanderson H, Kennedy J, Ritchie P, Goodwin G 2000 People plans and possibilities; exploring person centred planning. SHS, Edinburgh

Skinner B F 1953 Science and human behaviour. MacMillan, New York

The National Health Service and Community Care Act 1989 HMSO, London

Wolfensberger W 1972 The principle of normalisation in human services. National Institute on Mental Retardation. Toronto, Canada

12 Valuing people: in conclusion

Brian Kay

OVERVIEW This final chapter attempts to draw together the various aspects of provision for people with learning disabilities that have been discussed in the earlier chapters.

INTRODUCTION Whether you have read this book methodically through, chapter by chapter, or are using it primarily for reference, dipping in and out as the need presents, it is clear that what is presented is a journey both through time and through development of thought and practice. There have been a number of themes:

- exploring the development of service provision
- the practice of providing services in terms of planning and monitoring
- the specialised needs of groups with additional needs such as mental ill-health or old age
- the ethics of studies and provision changes
- exploring the often underestimated aspects of spirituality and ethical implications.

All these themes have centred around movement to a person-centred approach, discussing its interpretation, its implementation, its problems and its successes. Some chapters have considered general service aspects, such as Chapter 9, covering planning and monitoring of care, while others have dealt with particular additional needs occurring in some of those with learning disabilities: mental health (Ch. 4), the elderly (Ch. 10). Still other chapters have considered the particular problems that this group of people can face with situations that are common to all in society, such as bereavement (Ch. 6), sexuality (Ch. 3) and spirituality (Ch. 2).

The preceding chapters in this book have set the scene well for anyone wishing to follow and understand the development towards a person-centred, planned approach. However, the chapters have, I believe, done much more than this.

The novel areas in the book and the areas that move the evolution of thought and practice from enthusiastic ideals (described in Ch. 11) into meaningful events and actions in everyday life are those chapters considering spirituality (Ch. 2), sexuality (Ch. 3) and personal expression (Chs 6 and 10). It has taken the full weight of the philosophical development described in Chapter 11 to enable people to recognise the right to a spiritual life for people with learning disabilities. In the UK, we have been slow to recognise this. It was not that people with learning disability were deprived of access to religion; most mental handicap hospitals had thriving church services in their recreation halls every Sunday. However, this, valuable and important as it was, is some distance from recognising the true meaning of spirituality and spiritual experiences in life and indeed from leading a spiritual life. What value will any person-centred plan have that does not recognise the centre of the person? A spiritual existence and a personal spirituality is part of the very essence of personhood, and to fail to recognise that is to fail to recognise the person at the centre. It must be acknowledged that identifying and meeting spiritual needs is exceedingly difficult and challenging, but to fail to try is inexcusable. One of the most central challenges facing us in the development of support to people with a learning disability is to address spirituality and to recognise its pre-eminence for anyone to lead a full and meaningful life. Because it is too difficult or too esoteric is not a satisfactory excuse for not addressing this aspect, and Chapter 2 is an excellent starting point and guide to that process.

Much has been written in recent years about sexuality and people with learning disabilities. A large proportion of this has been on very pragmatic issues such as sexual health education, safe sex and more recently on the implications of sexually transmitted infections, including the human immunodeficiency virus (HIV) and the development of the acquired immunodeficiency syndrome (AIDS). All of these issues are important. Once it was finally established in our rights-based philosophy that people with a learning disability have similar sexual needs and feelings to the rest of society, and a perfect right to express and meet those needs, a huge leap was made in understanding and recognition. However, the practicalities of translating this recognition into a means of supporting people with learning disabilities in this aspect of their lives, on their terms, and respecting their aspirations, have proved far more challenging. This is one of the more difficult challenges to respond to for a number of reasons. First, it invariably involves more people than just the individual with the learning disability; second, there may well be a specific role for a 'professional' to offer guidance as well as support, at least in some aspects. It is an enormous challenge to bridge that particular gap and to be both supporter and advisor. John Stagg in Chapter 3 has given some extremely useful examples of how this can be approached and achieved. It is fascinating to try and meld the concepts of sexuality, sexual expression and spirituality together. Does some aspect of spirituality include concepts of morality? If we are to lead a spiritual life, are we also to lead a moral life? While we must recognise the norms of our society, not to mention the law and legalities, how does this impose upon our expression of our sexuality and our sexual aspirations? If we all have difficulties with such dilemmas, and I am sure most of us do, how are people with learning disabilities to be supported effectively in these aspects of their lives? Sadly, no book, even one as erudite as this one, is going to supply all the answers. However, it is imperative that we pose the questions and that we undertake the debate and explore the issues sensitively and seriously. The chapters in this book have all greatly added to this process.

The book has explored aspects of learning disability in the context of how we might perceive the nature of the disability itself. It has endeavoured to focus on the personhood of the individual and to relate the experience of learning disability to every aspect of 'normal' life. However, the preceding chapters have also addressed some of the divergences from our ordinary life model. These are not, per se, divergences from normality but rather from our expectations of normality. Consequently, one of the most powerful chapters is on mental health and learning disabilities (Ch. 4). Many (if not all) of us will at some time in our lives experience some form of mental ill-health. Whether it be the natural reaction to bereavement through loss of a close relative or friend, anxiety at a particularly challenging event or just the overwhelming stress of an aspect of our life that is beyond our control, we will all struggle to cope at one time or another. It is important to recognise that people with learning disabilities will experience this, just as other members of society do. As Chapter 4 shows, the development of this recognition and of the context in which mental health has been seen in relation to learning disabilities has been complex and not without controversy. As has been pointed out, mental health challenges have often been overlooked or misunderstood in the context of learning disability. Indeed, since, historically, learning disability was seen as a branch of psychiatry, much confusion has been generated. In addition, some of the professional agendas explored in Chapter 11 have had direct implications for how mental health has been understood and responded to. Some debates continue: for example, should people with learning disabilities be included in mental health legislation? This debate, which is a key component of Chapter 4, reflects the discussion in Chapter 11, which is that many of the considerations in the area of learning disability are as much political issues as social or philosophical ones. Hopefully, the person-centred approach will encourage much greater focus on supporting the individual, regardless of the aspect of their life for which they are seeking support. It should be possible to make a sensitive and effective response in the context of health needs and psychological well-being just as in any other aspect of everyday life. Again, this aspect of need may well require some 'professional' support, relying as it may on very specific experience, knowledge and expertise. However, as with the other areas explored in this book, it is the context in which support is sought and given that is paramount.

It is, perhaps, in the context of the out of the ordinary aspects of life that the application of the person-centred approach and our models of disability and autonomy are most challenged. Mental ill-health is a challenge for all, whether experiencing it or offering support. *Valuing people* (Department of Health, 2001) suggests that some people may have learning disabilities as part of additional challenges; for example, those who fall within the autistic spectrum disorders may have some degree of learning disability and may also experience difficulties in expressing their needs and aspirations. Indeed, they may have aspirations that it is difficult for society to respond to or meet.

CONCLUSIONS Finally, we consider the focus of this book. The issues explored are of relevance to all in society but particularly to people involved in any way in supporting those with learning disabilities, whether they be professionals, relatives, carers, advocates or interested parties, and to people with learning disabilities themselves (although not all the language used may have been as straightforward and jargon free as it could be). Inevitably, a significant part of our target audience will be those involved in service development and service provision; this is why, in addition to all the other aspects, the preceding chapters have also very specifically explored education and in particular the way in which professional education has developed and is provided. If we are to sustain the approaches and models we have identified here and if we are to meet, at last, the objectives of *Valuing people* (Department of Health, 2001) and a person-centred approach, then it is vital that those involved in providing support, care and services are educated and prepared in the right way. They will then be stimulated to join the debates necessary to broaden understanding and will develop the ability to make a useful and effective contribution to the process.

If this book contributes, even in a small way, to that process then it will have achieved the aspirations of its contributors and will have added to the steady growth and evolution of a positive approach to under-standing and meeting the needs of people with learning disabilities.

REFERENCES   Department of Health 2001 Valuing people: a new strategy for learning disability for the 21st century (Cm 5086). The Stationery Office, London

Index